Survival Skills for Pilates Teachers

Thriving in the mind-body fitness world

Nicola Conraths-Lange

Logokinesis Publishing • Ann Arbor

Logokinesis

Published by:

Logokinesis Publishing
805 Third Street
Ann Arbor, MI 48103
USA
info@logokinesis.com
www.logokinesis.com

Cover Photo:
© Jens Lange, 2003: "Saw on the Waterberg," Namibia, Africa, May 2003

Comics:
© Susan Byrnes, 2004

Cover and book design:
Holly Furgason, Interkinetic Creative Group

Printers:
Edwards Brothers, Ann Arbor, MI

Only what you share is yours forever.

From the Motion Picture *Monsieur Ibrahim*

About This Book

"Niki's book goes beyond the practice of bodywork and looks deep into the practitioner, uncovering many truths. This book's ability to heighten the practitioner's awareness, mixed with her wit, makes for a great read."

Brent D. Anderson, P.T., O.C.S., CEO of Polestar Education

"Whichever way you choose to use this book, USE IT. Let it become the bible in the midst of your Pilates books. Buy copies for friends and family. This book must be read! Thank you Niki for writing it."

Carolyne Anthony, Director of The Center for Women's Fitness

"Niki has written the book that has been in my head for seven years, but she has done the research, travel, and investigation necessary to make it so much more than an idea! This book is truly for everyone, because if you are not working in the mind-body fitness field, you are somewhere in your personal journey to mind or body fitness."

Nancy Hodari, Director of Equilibrium Fitness

"We all need Survival Skills! I applaud Niki's brave and ground-breaking endeavour to take on this monumental task. As a global community moving into the millennium, we need to adapt to a new world order. At the same time we must embrace and preserve the legacy of Joseph Pilates and the gift of his work, despite the immensely different environment in which we are surviving. This book serves as a guiding light for students and teachers of Pilates and mind-body fitness in general. The key to the survival and perpetuation of Pilates, with the integrity it was intended, is cooperation and collaboration. This is the essence of survival not only for teachers—but for humankind."

Rael Isacowitz, Founder and Director of Body Arts and Science International

"Niki Conraths' book is suffused with her enthusiasm for the art of teaching Pilates. Instructors will find a compassionate advocate in "Survival Skills for Pilates Teachers: Thriving in the Mind-Body Fitness World."

Elizabeth Larkam, Director of Pilates & Beyond

"Finally a book that speaks to the teacher and to the new teachers just entering the market. A must for every teacher to read."

Troy W. McCarty, Owner and Director of White Cloud Studios

"Niki Conraths' book Survival Skills for Pilates Teachers serves as a useful handbook for Pilates teachers. This is a resource that provides guidance for personal and professional development."

Trent McEntire, Program Director of McEntire Workout Method

"Survival Skills for Pilates Teachers offers a wealth of insight into the art & science of teaching Pilates."

Lindsay and Moira Merrithew, Co-founders of Stott Pilates

"Dieses Buch ist an all diejenigen gerichtet, die mit Menschen arbeiten, Feldenkrais-, Alexander- und PilateslehrerInnen. Die Vielfalt der Themen ist fantastisch."

[This book is directed toward any individual who works with people on a daily basis: Feldenkrais and Alexander practitioners as well as Pilates teachers. The breadth of the themes covered in this book is fantastic.]

Kornelia Ritterpusch, Owner of Studio für Körperbewusstsein

"Across the world of Pilates you can almost hear the collective sigh of relief. At last a book which tackles not whether you should zip or draw navel to spine, pelvic floor or no pelvic floor, turned in or turned out, but rather how to survive teaching Pilates! Teachers can now share the experience of other teachers and appreciate that they are not alone. I believe this book will also be relevant to other health and fitness practitioners. Well done Niki—I will be first in the queue to order my copy."

Lynne Robinson, Founder of Body Control Pilates

"Niki has a unique way of training and communicating. She is a true global ambassador for Pilates. The infectious enthusiasm which I experienced as her client can be found in every page of this book. Enjoy it!"

John Sealey, Communication Coach and Trainer

"We can only guide people on their journey as far and as deep as we ourselves have travelled. This book is an essential resource for any mind-body practitioner who is serious about the growth and embodiment of his or her profession. This book challenges our beliefs, boundaries, and sense of community within our professions and shares the 'Hows' of the journey."

Khita Whyatt, Director of Core Grace Pilates

Survival Skills for Pilates Teachers:
Thriving in the Mind-Body Fitness World

Nicola Conraths-Lange

Disclaimer:

Because there is always some risk involved, the author/publisher specifically disclaims any liability, loss, or damage caused or alleged to be caused by this book and accepts no responsibility for omissions or inaccuracies in this book. This includes any adverse effects or consequences resulting from suggestions, procedures, and preparations in this book. Please do not use the book if you are unwilling to assume the risk. Consult your physician or health professional before starting any type of physical activity.

Trademarks in this book are used under license:

Body Arts and Science International™

Body Control Pilates®

Franklin Method™

GYROTONIC®

Logokinesis™

McEntire Workout Method™

Pilates Method Alliance®

PMA™

Polestar Pilates Education™

STOTT PILATES® is a registered trademark of the Merrithew Corporation

Contents

About the Author

Foreword

Introduction

References

Acknowledgment

Contact Information

About the Author

Niki Conraths-Lange was born "feet first" and always wanted to dance. She sees herself as a global nomad, following her parents from Geneva, Switzerland, to Rome, Italy, where she grew up, and later to London, England, where she completed her dance studies.

After a few years of performing with several dance companies and independent projects, she suffered a severe lower back injury that brought her career to an abrupt stop. For the better part of one year, she had to look at the world from a supine position, wondering what on earth she was going to do with her life devoid of her lifelong passion: dancing.

After going through conventional rehab and regaining some control over her back and legs, she embarked on an exciting venture as an event manager. She toured through Europe with rock groups such as the Rolling Stones, Bon Jovi, Janet Jackson, and Phil Collins, utilizing her language and organizational skills.

But something was missing! After meeting her future husband, Jens, she took a leap into a new life and moved to the United States where she avidly pursued a bachelor's degree and then a master's degree in communication. At the same time, Pilates came into her life, and amazed at the wonderful impact it had on her still-hurting body, she decided to certify as a Stott Pilates instructor.

Since then, Niki has opened a successful studio in Hamburg, Germany. She specializes in the communication aspect of movement-related activities. Her company, Logokinesis, offers workshops and teaching advice for trainers.

Niki is on the Dance and Pilates faculty at Wayne State University, and she is currently completing her dissertation in Performing Arts Studies at Brunel University, London. She keeps herself happily busy presenting at national and international dance medicine and Pilates conferences, teaching at her studio in Ann Arbor, and attempting to sail the Great Lakes on her husband's wooden boat. The dance goes on!

Artist Susan Byrnes is a sculptor, painter, and photographer from upstate New York. Susan holds a BFA from Syracuse University and just completed her MFA in sculpture. Her work has been featured in numerous galleries from New York to Chicago. She was the executive director of the Peter Sparling Dance Company for 4 years and got in touch with Pilates during that time. She thinks we are all mad and talk about it too much, but she loves us nevertheless! Her award-winning, humorous sketches capture those situations that only trainers can understand—they will brighten your day.

Foreword

When Niki first started asking me questions about my life and teaching, I didn't pay too much attention. It was only when her questions started to make me think a little and ponder my life as a trainer that I finally asked her what she was up to.

"Writing a book," she said nonchalantly.

What a book this has turned out to be. She has taken all the questions we as trainers have asked ourselves, and she has given us the answers. She has analyzed them and given them structure and credence. With this book, she has enabled us to organize our lives to be more efficient at what we do and to spend some time nurturing ourselves.

Niki's book has made me step back and take a good long look at not just my teaching but also at how it affects my relationship with my husband and children. I am now able to not only recognize what I am doing wrong but to rectify it.

For me personally, it was a relief to know other trainers felt the way I did. I was not alone. Others had this love/hate relationship with the one thing that we are all passionate about—helping people discover the wonder of their bodies.

This book is filled with humor (the chapter on anatomy had me using my TA muscles!) and gets to the point, but it is compassionate, and above all, it is about real people in real situations. Niki then takes it one step further and gives us real solutions. After reading the book,

I have implemented some of what she has suggested, and it truly works. My business is much more focused. I refer clients who don't suit my way of teaching to others knowing that in no way does it mean I am not good enough. What a relief; I honestly thought I should be able to accommodate everyone.

Niki suggests that during our training as Pilates instructors we get a section on how to actually survive the life as a trainer. I couldn't agree with her more. This book will be required reading for all my students, and I encourage other organizations to do the same. For the real teachers out there, this will be a tool to help them in their life-long pursuit toward excellent teaching. For the undecided, it may serve as a reality check.

This book will also find its way to my husband's bedside table. This will be in the bedroom that is now painted a soothing sage green, with candles for lighting, soft music playing, and maybe a couple of cats purring on the bed.

Whichever way you choose to use this book, USE IT. Let it become the bible in the midst of your Pilates books. Buy copies for friends and family.

This book must be read.

Thank you, Niki, for writing it.

Carolyne Anthony

The Center for Women's Fitness, Ann Arbor, Michigan

Introduction

I longed for a philosophy, an all-embracing approach, a better way to explain to clients, family, and friends why movement needs to be part of our lives.

I longed for a forum of likeminded people who would be willing to bring the benefits of mind-body fitness to every area of our lives such as schools, hospitals, senior centers, and universities.

I also longed for continuing education models that cherish the element of community as opposed to competition, emphasizing the value of our life experiences to bring texture to the profession.

Are you of a like mind?

We all long for inspiration. At the last Body Mind Spirit conference in Santa Clara, which grouped together 1,200 attendees and an impressive array of top presenters, I experienced presentations by thirty extremely knowledgeable, well-known mind-body practitioners. All of them were interesting and had a lot to offer.

The thoughts of two of them I will take with me forever.

Why? Because they had pathos, they were emotional; they provided inspiration that went well beyond technical components of an exercise. I cried and felt connected. For a brief moment, I was a human being, not a human doing.

I wrote this book because I needed help. There were no books to advise me on the many things that I had questions about after I started teaching. So I asked other teachers who were more experienced than I was and realized the wealth of information that is out there but hard to get to.

It seemed we were all thinking the same thing: Teaching Pilates is great, but how do you handle everything it involves? The people, the business, our health. . .?

So the idea for a book was born. I slowly worked my way forward by attending conferences, speaking to so many of you, and approaching those who lead our field, "the teachers' teachers," so to speak, for advice. The result of this 18-month project is in your hands right now. Please help me make it better.

If I "hit the nail on the head" and parts of this book make you laugh or cry or make you think, "Yes that's me!" please get in touch. If you have more stories, if I missed something really important, if I made you mad with some of my comments, or if I got it totally wrong, call it out and email me. I will save every snippet of information for the next edition, so that this book will truly reflect all of our voices.

I cannot wait to hear from you!

Niki Conraths-Lange

1

Your Pilates Philosophy

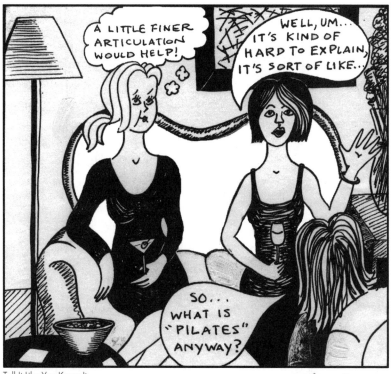

Tell It Like You Know It

Think about what Pilates, yoga, or Gyrotonic could bring to our sedentary world if they were everyday activities in our schools and workplaces. Let me paint this image of mind-body awareness just for one moment—it is too nice a thought to give up.

Relaxation Is Part of Life

Children today have never been busier. In the United States, many youngsters have tighter schedules than top managers do. Few children play on the street in front of their houses anymore; now they go abroad, take lessons, travel on teams, and are often tired. On the other side of the spectrum, the impact of technology is becoming noticeable in the younger generation. Susanne Martin, a physical therapist and author from California, is seeing a lot of keyboard-related posture problems in her practice. Adults today started becoming computer literate a lot later than young children, the repercussions of which are yet to be seen. Even in Japan, (the land of Zen. . .), many high achievers are suffering from academic burnout syndrome.

How would a daily practice of Pilates, yoga, or Gyrotonic influence the coming generation? I would argue that, biomechanical issues aside, such practices could offer them a lifelong tool for energizing themselves in stressful times and a forum for communion in their families and workplaces. As such, one of the missions of Pilates practitioners could be to reach out and teach the young generation much more actively.

Body and Mind Go Together

Body-mind practices teach us that we should honor the shell as much as the brain, because the two entities are incomplete when out of balance. Mind-body awareness is a powerful gauge for how far we can push ourselves without creating irreversible damage. Sometimes a person will walk into the studio and tell his story of "living with pain": pain standing up, pain sitting down; pain lifting an arm, pain climbing the stairs. And yet, he keeps going, doing what he does, until he cannot take it any longer.

Carol Davis, keynote speaker at the Polestar conference in Miami, is a scholar and author that has been researching empathy for years. She touched on the drama inherent in such a lifestyle: "No human should wake up thinking that they are not able to face the day," she says. "Flowers don't do it; animals don't do it."

How can the threshold of bearable pain be endured for so long, when it impacts our quality of living and our relationships, and effectively rules every aspect of our lives? For one, we are trained to ignore our bodies right from the very start: at school, we are taught to sit still and concentrate. Therefore, in our minds, "important things," things that require concentration and alertness, are associated with "non-movement."

The reality is different: the body needs to be active, needs to use breath, needs stretching, needs cardiovascular activity. Even the most domesticated animal will not just get up and go without stretching UNLESS there is a dramatic reason that calls for immediate alertness and attention, such as defending its territory or pursuing food.

By watching animals, sedentary and non-active people can quickly understand what the Pilates "hype" is all about. Animals stretch with so much gusto and joy that I wonder two things when watching human runners (probably the world's worst stretchers) contorting themselves by craning their legs up onto a high surface, with misaligned pelvis and distorted hips:

1. What exactly do they think they are stretching?

2. Why do they look so tensed and upset while doing this, when it is obviously not stretching any of the muscle groups that could legitimately cause such anguish?

Joy of movement is important. Feeling a great stretch, a release in the hip joint or a gentle traction of the back is pure joy! Valuing the element of concentration linked to intelligent movement is joyful. Lying down in the constructive rest position itself can be a philosophical exercise, can it not?

I miss it when I go a day without consciously lying down, feeling my spine, checking in with my alignment. Imagine, some people NEVER lie down on the floor. NEVER!

Wellness Boom

After the group aerobic wave of the 1980's, in which working out was a communal affair and had to involve cardiovascular activity, the 1990's changed our approach to fitness: we wanted to balance, not just build muscle, we needed calm and quiet to juxtapose our hectic work schedules, and we discovered "homemade" wellness that was suddenly accessible to all social classes and not just reserved for the Hollywood stars.

The stores are full of aromatherapy oils for home use, salts and creams, massage balls, yoga mats, eye pillows—many things that were definitely not mainstream just a few years ago. Pampering yourself is ok, in fact it is finally making its way into our lives as a necessity and not perceived as something warranting a guilt trip. Hurray!!

As usual, there are a lot of scams out there: yogis who want to make fast cash opening yoga studios, Pilates teachers who buy a $39.95 certification package over the Internet, and some Instructor who just learn the method from a book. Poor clients!

The mind-body boom has catapulted the Pilates method to the forefront of a fast-growing industry. The Pilates Method Alliance, a not-for-profit professional organization dedicated to preserving the work of Joseph and Clara Pilates, estimated that in the year 2000, 1.7 million Americans were exposed to Pilates lessons. In 2001, this number grew to 2.4 million, and in 2002, an amazing 4.7 million Americans have been exposed to the method either through videos, their local gyms, or trying a Pilates class as a result of a magazine or newspaper article. Five million people already.

Pilates has become synonym for lifestyle, so much so that there is now even a magazine out, "Pilates Style." They claim that not five million people are doing Pilates but twelve. I cannot wait until we make it into the White house. . .

When I certified, I knew breaths and modifications on all the required exercises and felt prepared and able to teach. The teaching, although a little rocky at first, went well. The daily encounter with people, their personalities, and their ups and downs, were aspects of teaching that I really enjoyed.

What caught me completely off guard were the cancellations, re-scheduling, late payments, and hours of phone calls per month in order to streamline my ever-changing schedules. When you work for a studio, those issues may seem trivial because a front desk takes care of them. When we have our own studios, however, and are called upon as managers, accountants, helpers, healers and cashiers, we have endless opportunity for huge mistakes. These are hard to rectify: once you have given one client a special rate or not charged a cancellation fee, you set a precedent. This whole money thing has been the source of much grief in my brief time as a Pilates practitioner.

Coming from an academic communication background, I started wondering about the lack of information regarding the soft skills in our job. There was no "getting started on the job" or "roadblocks and pitfalls in the life of a Pilates trainer" section in the manual. All things considered, I would say that choosing Pilates as a career is hugely rewarding.

Pilates teachers meet people from different cultures and backgrounds in a non-threatening environment which is aimed at improving their body awareness, health, and enjoyment for movement. Oftentimes we are the "highlight" of their week and after class, they leave energized and "on top of the world." How amazing is it to be the person that people look forward to seeing? And how proud are we when our clients make progress, attempting exercises that a few months ago may have seemed impossible?

And still, I also believe that we can only "give" well and appropriately to others, if we know how to take care of ourselves. At the beginning, all we can think of is getting busy and teaching all day long. Then we slowly start to experience the other things: dealing with clients, no time to work out ourselves, no time for family and friends, and possibly even injuries, that may result from non-ergonomic teaching practices. We must apply the same standards that we set for our clients to ourselves:

1. Find time to relax.

2. Make time for your own workouts regularly.

3. Listen to your body.

Do we do it?

What role would we want a certifying organization to assume, if we determined that it would be useful to cover such areas in the curriculum, or if these were offered as continuing education modules?

Dear Pilates organizations, the people you certify, if mentored and developed, will be your loyal and loving backbone when times get rough! We will keep our studios going and the integrity of the method intact because you made an effort to prepare us for the job ahead. Here are some questions that may be worth asking of your students:

1. Teaching

    a   Why do you want to be a Pilates teacher?

    b   Do you just like doing Pilates or are you genuinely interested in imparting knowledge as an educator?

The two talents of moving well and teaching well can be at opposite sides of the personal spectrum. The love of movement has performing aspects to it, which are to some extent egocentric. Teaching, on the other hand, is probably the most altruistic profession there is. How do we marry the two?

When we work, we don't DO Pilates to others. We TEACH Pilates. The doing is a private matter. The teaching is a vocation, but it also requires skills that can be learned and perfected. The best way to witness teaching is by means of apprenticeship and mentorship. Watching a teacher who has a vocation for teaching will teach us many of the skills we need to be able to work as Pilates teachers for a very long time with enthusiasm and cachet.

Vocation comes from the Latin word "vocare" which means a "calling." It implies a higher belief system, and has an almost religious connotation. The reason I bring this up is because men and women with a calling have boundless energy. Rael Isacowitz, founder of Body Arts and Science International, is a prime example of this type of teacher. He is so passionate about what he does that he is able to summon unknown reserves of power and energy that are difficult to match. Are we able to summon that kind of energy every day?

Let us consider career questions within Pilates.

2. Career

   a Do you see yourself teaching in a gym, a Pilates studio, or on your own?

   b If you do not want to open your own studio, can you see yourself running around town teaching at a million places when you are in your 50's?

There are so many aptitude tests out there that could be adapted for our job so that we could be guided in a good direction depending on our personalities and interests. A twenty-year ongoing study from the business school of Wayne State University shows clearly that the number-one reason why small businesses fail is related to the owners' characteristics. We have to take our personalities into account when determining where we want to go with Pilates and where our talents will work best.

Identifying our strengths is important in order to avoid burnout later on. In our line of work, where energy is not just drained from the sheer physical activity of teaching but also from constant human interaction, the right workplace is key. Choosing our workplace wisely, with our personality needs in mind, is important for our mental and physical health. Why teach in a studio if we like the buzz of a gym? Why teach in people's homes if we do not like to drive? Identifying our needs should be part of the education process of becoming a teacher. We can only work at our best if we feel safe and valued. The process of identifying the where, when, and how demands our thoughts and attention.

Bits and Pieces

There are also many other less crucial issues that would be good to ask questions about in instructor training. Communication skills are very important because teaching mat classes in a group setting with more temporary clients requires different skills from teaching and retaining private clients over several years. Buying equipment requires making choices about what we need and how our budgets figure in to the equation. Last but not least, organizational elements such as drafting and implementing policies in our workplaces and with our clients are harder than we think.

No matter how popular Pilates will become in the future, nobody will pay between $60 and $120 and hour "just" for exercises. As trainers we must have knowledge, for sure, but also sensitivity and a philosophy. This includes knowing when you are not the right person to work with a specific individual.

A good plan should be linked to a philosophy. All that this means is that we should think about, question, and frame our approach to the work. In academia, they call this a "theoretical framework." A framework establishes where we come from in terms of beliefs and approach to the world. For example: are you someone who believes that our life is in our hands and that we have a big stake in what happens to us? Or do you believe in a more fatalistic approach to life, in which our paths are pre-established by a higher entity? Sometimes your philosophy is linked to your religion. Other times life happenings make you change your philosophy.

Brent Anderson, CEO of Polestar, verbalized his philosophy during a workshop. Anybody who attended the class with me will confirm that it was a special kind of class in more ways than one. Brent taught us a mat class. The class had a lot of good information, had excellent flow, and was funny as well. What made it special, though, was his closing statement: Brent believes that Pilates practice improves the quality of living of those who subscribe to it. He is adamant about the fact that mind-body fitness makes a difference in people's lives by fostering understanding and respect of other human beings. Pilates could therefore possibly reduce abuse in our families and communities. It can make us happier, more fulfilled people. He calls it "impacting the world through intelligent movement" as described in his company's mission statement.

He also has some really good arguments to back this up: we teach "important" people: dignitaries, government officials, top managers, judges, even presidents. And due to the nature of our work, we are darn close to them! Maybe from now on, the saying that there is a great woman behind every great man will change to: there is a Pilates teacher behind every great man and woman.

It was one of those "magical" moments of direction and leadership. Brent cried, we all cried. Fabulous!

Note how his philosophy encompasses different methods or labels. It simply states that doing Pilates has positive outcomes for our social relationships, teaches us respect for ourselves, and therefore makes it easier to respect others. "I think I have more empathy for others since I started doing yoga," my mother, who never exercised until well into her 50's, told me other day. I was amazed at her comments and surprised at the far-reaching consequences this entailed.

Knowing and stating our philosophy will drive us to the types of clients with whom we will be most successful in working. If you believe that body and mind work together and that there is no healing of one entity without including the other in the process, you will be unhappy working with individuals who use Pilates as a method of exercise to lose weight for purely aesthetic reasons or shape their bodies in predetermined ways.

Conversely, a client who comes to you and expects psychological counseling along with Pilates training and is used to a cosmic, all-encompassing teaching approach will be running away from you if all you talk about is muscles: lines of energy are this person's philosophy.

Clients now look for a place to relax and recharge—the trainer and the studio environment are the key facets that speak to one individual, while making the next one feel ill at ease. Personality and the ability of a trainer to verbalize his or her philosophy and approach to the work are essential elements for making a trainer credible and justifying ethical standards that he or she sets in place.

Verbalizing Your Philosophy

In this society, public speaking and good argumentation skills are identified with intelligence and capability. There may be many fantastic therapists out there who are having a hard time staying afloat due to poor verbalization and marketing skills. How would you feel if you called up a chiropractor and he said: "Ahem, uh, well we sort of make you straight again by cracking your bones"?

These skills are not rocket science; they can be learned!

So let's start with assessing the status quo. What is the essence of Pilates from your perspective? Take a few moments to describe what Pilates IS and what Pilates is NOT. The following is my list of the "is" and "is not" of Pilates.

Pilates IS:	Pilates is NOT:
An Exercise Method	A Team sport
A Philosophy	A Trend
Strengthening	Weight Management
Balancing	Competitive
Mindful	Repetitive or Fast
Anaerobic	Aerobic
Articulating/Isotonic	Isometric
A constant in your life	An occasional affair

Let's just be clear on what it is that we do, instead of responding negatively to denying people's perceptions. Most people will have read about the new trend of Pilates in a magazine. They believe that this is some new gadget that they need to check out. Wrong. Pilates has been around for a very long time, almost a hundred years, and has a legacy to it. Length of time establishes credibility, especially for methods that claim to produce change in the body, let alone in the mind. So, when you describe Pilates, the following formula works best:

1. How long has it been around? Who was Joseph Pilates?

The name Pilates refers to the late Joseph Pilates who was born in 1880. He was a sickly child and conditioned himself to become and accomplished boxer and circus performer through his own method of rehabilitation, which was later tested in English war prisoner camps. He was one the first to combine the elements of Eastern philosophies with Western ideas of fitness. Pilates immigrated to the United States from Germany in the 1950's and opened a studio in New York City that was frequented by many dancers, actors, and Hollywood stars. The Pilates we teach today is based on his principles, but includes medical knowledge on body mechanics and rehabilitation that has been developed after his death.

2. What IS it?

Pilates is a method of exercise that is based on a body-mind philosophy. This approach is based on the belief that our wellbeing and health originate from a stable core (our centers) that supports our skeleton and allows joints and muscles to be balanced. Balance can be achieved by mindful movement, limited repetitions of a given exercise, and the integration of breath. Pilates will help you with balance, the state of peaceful strength of being in the moment that requires optimal interplay of strength and flexibility. A repertory of over 500 exercises on different pieces of equipment and on the mat is available for a lifetime of challenge and growth. Pilates is a choice, and its principles will influence any other type of activity you will pursue. It is a foundation for the way you see your body and the world.

3. What is it NOT?

Pilates is not a trend or a machine. It will not make you loose weight or show fast results if done inconsistently. It is not fundamentally aerobic, although in advanced stages it can be, and it is not performed while watching TV, reading a magazine, or talking on the phone. It does not randomly build muscle and is not a group sport. It is not competitive.

Practice your Pilates philosophy statement over and over again with a different focus. Do you require a quick sentence or a more in-depth description? Is the person you are talking to truly interested, or are you just making conversation at a party? Keep it simple and consider your audience: there is nothing worse than asking an engineer a polite "So what do you do?" and being stuck with him for two hours faking interest about auto parts. (I live in Motown, it happens a lot.)

People are bombarded with snippets of information that do not necessarily make sense, because the journalists writing them probably have not taken a Pilates class before. Following are quotes that I have gathered in the media, on the Internet, in newspapers, and in books:

- Pilates will change your life
- Pilates will make you feel revitalized and confident, and improves your posture
- Pilates is good for you
- Pilates trains your body awareness

All these statements are true, but where is the argument behind them? Where is the logical train of thought that makes clients realize that there is potential for truth in these statements?

Becoming a Fine Oriental Rug

We have to think about what we say and know what we mean. My visual explanation for the benefits of Pilates is a fine oriental rug. In Istanbul, when you visit the bazaar, making rugs is just as much a science as an art. A fine rug boasts several thousands of hand-knitted knots per square inch. The knots have to be perfectly aligned and as close as possible to the previous knots. Oftentimes the weaver has to undo them and start again until the intricate patterns are perfect.

The more knots there are, the more valuable the rug becomes. Its colors will be vibrant and ever-changing depending on the orientation of the fibers. You can run your hand across these masterpieces and marvel at their texture and softness. All this work does not only make them beautiful. The rugs are durable and resistant to the elements. You can empty a whole bottle of wine or olive oil on a fine rug and just brush it off.

Every hour we spend schooling awareness, realizing the endless capabilities of our bodies when we put our minds to it, are hand-knitted knots. They become the texture of our being and gently weave through our bodily shells. We hand-make our own Oriental rug bodies. We know how we got through a certain movement or exercise every step of the way. We call it building strength, but it really is much more powerful than that. This kind of approach gives us the same control over life's mishaps that the weaver has over flaws in the rug; we can undo mistakes and start again so that our bodies and our minds become stronger and more integrated."

When my lower back injury was at its worst, my life became a scary place. It was not a question of not being fit. I knew that I was millions of miles away from fitness. It was different; I felt like a ghost. The smallest thing could knock me over: people, cars, stairs. I did not even have the strength to stand my own ground as a human being. I had turned into an old bathroom mat. That's exactly how I felt!

My ordeal lasted for about ten months. Ten months of agony due to a weakened, inexistent body-mass. This experience I will never forget, and it is one of the main reasons why I chose to teach Pilates. It has given me my life back. A life in which I cannot only move from point A to point B without pain, but a life that enables me to travel and—most importantly—dance again. A life that gives me the opportunity to work and understand others who are in the same situation now, and really know what they are going through.

Sometimes we are put on the spot by people asking questions about what Pilates is all about. We are asked to reduce a philosophy into concepts that are totally meaningless such as "tight abs" and "toned arms." That is just not enough for us to wake up in the mornings and look forward to a day in the studio.

Our philosophy is the spine of our work. It should be strong but flexible, articulate yet connected. Our philosophy can be extended if we care to reach for the stars, or it can be articulate and detailed if we choose to glance at the world upside down, to make new sense of it.

We shape our own reality.

2

Being a Pilatista:
What It Takes, How We Get It!

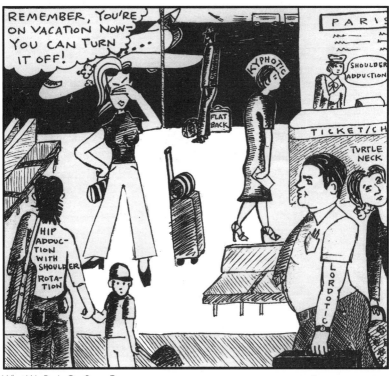

What We Do In Our Spare Time

coined the term "Pilatista" with friends on a warm summer evening in Rome. The ending "ista" has Spanish and Italian roots, and is slowly making its way into mainstream conversational English. A "fashionista," for example, is "someone who can stumble out of a swamp covered with leeches and still look like a million bucks," according to an article that appeared in the Denver Rocky Mountain News (of all places).

Being a Pilatista is not just a hobby or something you undertake on a whim. "Istas" are proud, passionate, and emotional about what they love. Being an "ista," to me, is a way of life; it describes people who enthusiastically support an art, trend, or method.

Pilates teachers love what they do so much that their jobs carry over to their personal lives and conversations all the time.

How many hours have I spent analyzing anatomical principles and how they relate to a client with my studio partner? How many more hours have I focused on discussing exercise modifications and their applicability in a mat or private class? How many thousands of hours have I spent trying to understand why some people in pain remain adamant about lifting heavy weights and running on a treadmill with bodies that, at best, should just lie down and breathe?

Sadly, I also have to admit that my friend Philip Madrid and I have had the audacity to spend two hours on the phone discussing the Psoas muscle. He lives in New Mexico; I live in Michigan.

Weird, I know, but we had a great time.

"Sometimes I see teachers talking about Pilates day and night, constantly, 'Should I turn it in or out, pointed or flexed,' and I just want to shout out loud: 'Get a life!'" says Lynne Robinson, director of Body Control Pilates in the UK. She is so right! I wish I could turn it off.

It seems to me that Pilates teachers like to spend time with other Pilates teachers. We don't run away from our coworkers when it is 5PM, and if we leave the job, never see them again. Many of my closest friends do what I do. The reason why it is so interesting to spend time with Pilatistas is that they have led such amazing lives.

Wanting to teach Pilates is not something we grow up with, like wanting to be a fireman or a ballerina. Teaching Pilates is something you get to—it's a journey. Many of us are dancers and have been seriously injured. Others are physical therapists or doctors discovering Pilates as a way to improve our practices. Others still were business people in need of a change, women who wanted a second career after their children grew up, and people who retired and teach Pilates to the passionate over 60's crowd that make up half of our studios' populations.

"Most Pilates teachers I have met are dancers," says George Evans, a long-term Pilates client. "And," he adds, "most of them were injured." Since dancers make up such a large part of the Pilates teaching population, it is widely assumed that they make good teachers. If we look at the previous jobs of the owners of Pilates organizations, there is a common theme with one exception:

Elizabeth Larkam: dancer

Moira Merrithew: dancer

Rael Isacowitz: dancer

Gordon Thompson: dancer

Alan Herdman: dancer

Brent Anderson: physical therapist (who dances. . .)

Well? Do dancers make the best teachers?

"Yes, without a doubt," say Eva Powers and Nancy Hodari, from the Stott Pilates certification center Equilibrium in Bloomfield Hills, Michigan.

"I can almost guarantee that dancers make fabulous instructors," says Nancy. "The dancers who have entered our program are consistently successful in achieving certification due in large part to their prior movement education that has required precision and discipline.

Because dancers understand movement, I see them looking at clients with so much interest. Trainees who are dancers never seem to experience frustration when dealing with the challenge of a rigorous training program. For dancers, Pilates is another form of movement, thus they never feel like they are strangers in a strange land. They study movement, they understand movement, they feel movement."

Eva Powers, professor of dance at Wayne State University and Stott instructor teacher, is of a like mind: "Dancers just have such an advantage due to their training. They are accustomed to cueing and have excellent body awareness and kinesthetic awareness."

Nancy also mentions the element of "flow," which is so important when performing the exercises. Flow refers to the artistry and quality of a movement, a notion that literally transforms dance, which could be functionally described as an amalgamation of movements on different planes, into what it is: an art form. Likewise, looking at Pilates from a more artistic, life-transforming, or healing angle is beneficial for all of us teaching it. If it is art, it is fresh and new every day.

Now, there is the other side of the coin. If you are thinking about pursuing certification and are not a dancer, there is no need to be discouraged. Lynne Robinson, founder of Body Control Pilates in the UK, literally fell into it and dragged her husband Leigh with her.

Lynne was a history teacher with terrible posture and a bad back. She admits to having very poor coordination skills. She could not lift her right arm and left leg simultaneously, she tells me, laughing at her beginnings.

"Gordon Thomson trained me to teach. I think it helped that I called him long distance from Australia and he couldn't see me. He may have changed his mind otherwise!" Lynne remembers. Gordon was Lynne's teacher and mentor, and they later went on to found Body Control Pilates.

Due to her Pilates life story, she has a different approach to certification and life in general than dancers do, which is just as artistic in a slightly different way.

"I think that dancers, which make up a large part of our teacher group, do not necessarily make the best teachers." Lynne says "They can perform the advanced work, sure. They look wonderful doing it and many are also very talented teachers. But being able to do the exercises well does not necessarily make you good at teaching them! We see the full mat as an end goal for our clients. But it is the journey there that matters. Many may not ever be able to do swan dive, but you don't need to be a concert pianist to enjoy and benefit from playing the piano! I think that that's why we have been so successful. We have broken down the original exercises and made Pilates accessible to everybody."

Lynne's unusual path to Pilates teaching influences the commitment of her company to invite people from all backgrounds to partake in teacher training programs. Of course, students with no previous education in fitness or movement are required to have a longer period of training and recommendations from an instructor. But, Lynne feels passionate about integrating people from all walks of life into her organization.

Are we dancers out of touch with the struggle that accompanies learning movement from scratch? Is our background so different? Do our bodies seem as if they were created on another planet from the population at large? I guess so. We can explain what an exercise is supposed to feel like, but we cannot feel what it is like never to have moved. How can we truly understand a body that is not accustomed to movement if we have never walked that path?

The only plausible answer to this is that we all have walked a difficult path at some point in time. We have experienced pain, joy, and frustration. We all have a common denominator that allows us to connect as human beings. This will help us connect with different kinds of clients.

We can all learn many exercises and be knowledgeable about

anatomy, but what truly makes us good teachers? Being an exceptional teacher requires a special connection with a special client. We are all exceptional for a special person. And they are the same to us. That is why everyone who is truly drawn to mind-body professions should really live them, no matter what background they come from.

Life Stories

Philip Madrid is one of those people who got into a profession he did not really like because it felt weird to him to do what he is passionate about. He is passionate about fitness, and always has been. He lifted weights for 15 years and read every book about nutrition, stretching, and muscle toning ever released. He spent whole days at the gym.

Phil also roamed the world for four years in the navy as a young man and then went on to engineering school. After he got his masters degree, a major U.S. car manufacture promptly hired him.

He quickly rose through the ranks but loathed his job. He had issues with his coworkers who thought he was eating strange foods (hummus, salads, and juices), and who thought it was weird that he did not own a house, or have two cats, a wife, or children. They were also probably intrigued and puzzled by the strange things he did in his free time. If they had visited his apartment, they would have been even more amazed. Way back then, he had no furniture except for body building equipment: equipment, and more equipment.

Nancy Hodari remembers when Phil's resume came to her attention. "When our education department at Equilibrium received Philip's application, they immediately put it on my desk," she says. "Our curiosity was at an all-time high: an automotive engineer, with a background in ballet, applying for full-time certification? For two years, we grew used to a man in a suit and briefcase arriving daily at around 6PM, and like Clark Kent, transforming himself from corporate mode to mind-body mode."

I had a similar experience. "Hi, my name is Phil. I would like to take ballet lessons to broaden my horizons," is what I heard when I picked up the phone four years ago.

This is how our communal journey started. For him, our friendship led him into a different career, since my Pilates-infused ballet lessons introduced him to the work. For me, it was amazing to see how a man who was unhappy in his profession became a fantastic teacher and mentor. Phil quit his high-paying job as an engineer to teach Pilates and Gyrotonic. He now holds more certifications than I can count and is especially good at working with young dancers and athletes. He pulls out the best in them and has even managed to adapt a Reformer made for adults to fit our six-year-old baby ballerina, Alexis.

Any regrets? "No way, I'll never go back," he says.

Peter Bowen and his wife Jan converted an old cart shed, made of Cheshire brick, into a Pilates studio. "We overlook farmland and see lots of wildlife," he writes.

This was quite a change from his former job, which involved planning airports.

This couple chose a radical career change and decided to do it together. They were both able to get an early retirement package, which was very helpful for setting up their business. Jan had had severe neck issues and was looking for something that could truly help her. Pilates was it. They probably never would have dreamt in their wildest dreams that the magazine "Your Horse" would do a feature article on their studio describing Equine Pilates. (This is Pilates for people who ride, not Pilates for horses!)

Some people also come from a total "body" background as dancers and decide to try a completely different path before they land on the Pilates shore. Jane Vatcher, a dancer from London, stunned us all when she told us that she was retiring from the stage eight years ago.

We could not believe it. Jane is one of those people who is born to perform; she absolutely loves the theater. But, London is a competitive place, and when she was in her early thirties, her favorite teacher and choreographer succumbed to AIDS. A whole generation of artists was left without leadership and inspiration. She just needed to get away from it all to grieve. Even staying in London, close to the performing buzz, was unbearable to her at the time.

Jane opened a vegetarian café on a Greek island called Symi and spent eight years there as a successful entrepreneur. She paid a price though: the job took its toll on her body. Standing for long sixteen hour days, washing up dishes, and preparing food was a lot to take. When I worked with her for the first time almost two years ago, a thigh stretch was so painful that it sent tears to her eyes—she had no idea that it had gotten so bad.

Jane loves Pilates and is now certified, back on her Greek island opening a Pilates and yoga retreat!

As you can see, our backgrounds are varied and so exciting! No wonder people like to spend time with us. But what are the skills that we need to be successful at what we do?

I asked many of my interviewees what they believe to be essential skills. It is quite a list.

1. Teachers must know the exercises and be able to apply modifications to clients' needs.

2. Teachers must have a working knowledge of anatomy from a functional perspective. Knowing muscles and their locations tells us nothing about how these translate into a human being with a specific posture.

3. Teachers need a "good eye." This refers to the ability to read muscular patterns across the body and subsequently being able to address problems at the "source." Everybody I spoke to agreed that this skill takes time.

4. Teachers need a social personality in order to be welcoming

and caring to many different people. If you are a loner, this job very well may not be your best bet.

5. A good teacher needs "empathy" more than "sympathy." Empathy allows us to identify with another person's feelings. Sympathy allows us to walk in someone else's shoes, recreating their feelings of anguish or joy in our own bodies. As practitioners, empathy is crucial; sympathy may make us too involved, and as a result, we lose objectivity and are less effective practitioners.

6. Teachers need to be articulate and clear. A warm tone of voice and musical phrasing of exercise cues are important.

7. Teachers are also role models. The ability to motivate clients, to be passionate about our work, and to be charismatic in some shape or form all play into the "practice what we preach" approach to teaching.

8. Teachers must be professional and follow standards of conduct. If we want to bend the rules, we should do so with awareness and good intentions.

9. Teachers should look tidy and neat, within the framework of their personalities. Being professional is somewhat reflected in the way we present ourselves.

10. Teachers should be aware of body odor. Believe it or not, this came up a lot. Using deodorant and brushing our teeth or having mints readily available makes our presence much more pleasant for our clients. (Note: This works in the reverse as well!)

Since Pilatistas come from so many different backgrounds and have made active choices to teach, the environment in which we will be able to shine and perform at our best is very important. We should start thinking about this right away during our training. Here are some options:

Gym or Athletic Club

A personal trainer in a gym or athletic club is usually certified in a variety of fitness activities. Due to the fast-paced, constantly changing fitness trends, an instructor at such a facility will work on many different pieces of equipment per day, depending on client demand and club schedule. Typically, they will see about three to four personal clients per day, then teach a step or aqua aerobics class, and after that they may teach a Pilates mat or stretch class. Gyms are busy places; they are often loud and crowded. Classes are made up of a core of steady clients and many others who will drop in. This creates a big imbalance in levels that you have to cater to.

The introspective element of Pilates has a hard time gaining momentum in a Gym environment. Barbara Basset, a trainer who predominantly teaches in an athletic club, put it this way: "I feel like a lot of my club clients don't want to listen. Many of them don't think it 'does' anything unless it's hard, unless you sweat, unless you are sore the next day. I feel like I have to feed them a candy bar filled with vitamins, yin and yang, a bit of both."

On the other hand, a gym or club has a broader fitness horizon, depending on our goals. If we want to provide a broad spectrum of training that includes cardiovascular and weight lifting activity, the gym is perfect.

If we like it more personable, warm, and small, working at a Pilates studio is our other option.

The Pilates Studio

Throughout my travels, I have had the opportunity to see many, many different Pilates studios in Germany, Italy, England, Spain, the US, South Africa, and Canada.

I absolutely love going to different studios and catching the "vibe." Some of them have really influenced the way I teach and how I set up my own studio, whereas in others I was flabbergasted, stared in awe, and knew that I could never afford such extravagant facilities.

A few of them just gave me the creeps!

Pilates studios try to create an atmosphere that encourages concentration, relaxation, and wellbeing. Sometimes, there will be soft background music, and often we see candles or incense burning. There may be photographs on the walls depicting models doing Pilates exercises or art that is soothing and peaceful.

The lighting is soft and warm (no neon), and high ceilings are preferable when possible.

My favorite studio in Germany had a kitchen with wellness teas or ginger water for clients, as well as offering a five-minute shiatsu massage at the end of the session (heaven!). There was nothing on the walls and a minimalist Japanese interior design characterized the room.

At any given time, there would be simultaneous classes going on, with up to five trainers working in a medium-sized room alongside a large mat class.

Unlike a gym, a Pilates studio generally has no membership dues. Although many studios offer standing mat or Reformer classes for groups, clients typically have to pre-register in order to guarantee a space. Since Pilates is about finding the right level for each person, open classes are divided into levels, and a trainer will redirect the client to another class if the trainer feels the client is potentially hurting himself or herself.

The downside of working in a studio is that you have a very heavy work schedule (just like in a gym), earn about half of what your client pays, and are usually asked to conform to a method that the studio endorses.

On the positive side, you have the tremendous benefit of getting to know many different body types in a short time, thereby building experience, you can watch experienced trainers, you do not have to worry about bookings, and you have access to all the equipment for working out yourself.

Relatively speaking, a studio is the perfect place for you if you like the atmosphere and your manager, you are happy leaving the negotiating and money matters to the front desk, and you just want to concentrate on teaching without the hassle of administration.

BUT, if you do not want the gym, feel unchallenged in a studio, and have plenty of ideas on how to do it better, then go solo.

Solo

Going solo is amazingly challenging and rewarding. It requires careful planning, strategic decision-making, and most importantly, good people to advise you on the business side of things. When you go solo, you have to make all decisions pertaining to your studio and teaching approach. On top of that you need to devise and lead your advertising campaigns (see the next chapter for advice).

If you have financial backing, one supported way of going solo is to open a licensed facility under the auspices of a well-known Pilates association.

Polestar, for example, took the German market by storm through the partnership of Brent Anderson, CEO of Polestar Education, and physiotherapist Alexander Bohlander. There are many advantages to opening a licensed facility. You can easily market the product because the name is established. You will be able to place your contact information on the company's Web site, which probably will get hundreds of hits per day. If you are a good negotiator, you can arrange special payment options for equipment and offer exclusive certification courses in a 300 mile radius.

Opening a licensed facility often requires you to be admitted to a special instructor trainer program in order to allow you to train others. You will probably have a jump start in terms of client demand, but you have to be able to meet the need; if you have too many requests, you will not be able to teach 15-hour days, so you have to hire trainers. All of a sudden, you are an employer with all the problems that arise from leading others in their careers!

If your licensed studio grows, the financial rewards can be very good, but you will spend most of your time ADMINISTRATING rather than TEACHING Pilates. Ask yourself a million times if that is what you want!

The other way of going solo is by starting a small studio for private and mat classes that bears your distinct signature. At the beginning, your studio is YOU.

It is unlikely that your growth will be disproportionably high; you can experiment a little and find a format that works for you. For example: I am not an evening person when it comes to teaching, learning, or doing any concentrated activity. Since most people work while I am at my "best" as a trainer, and therefore they tend to gravitate toward evening courses or weekend classes, they "hit" me at a time when I do not have the amount of energy that is required to run a successful one-woman show.

So I established a format that worked with my personality: I started very early, sometimes at 6AM, and catered to high-earning, busy professionals who are on a plane or in meetings all day long and have dinners at night.

Their only chance for a workout is early in the mornings. They want to have private lessons because they are surrounded by people all day long and seldom have time for themselves. These relationships were immensely rewarding, because client need and trainer availability merged perfectly. My income for the day was basically set by 12PM.

This does not work for everybody, but a critical component of running a successful Pilates studio is knowing when you are at your best, which populations benefit most from your expertise, and when you should not be working because it is bad marketing.

At the end of the day, I decided that "soloing" was not for me. I wanted to do other things, such as write this book, so: Know when to shine, know when to decline!

An additional, very ambitious option within the realm of soloing is to develop your own approach to exercise with the intent to eventually become a large certifying organization. Trent McEntire, one of the first teachers at Equilibrium, decided to venture down this road less traveled after he had worked as an instructor teacher for Stott Pilates for several years. "I just felt that I had many ideas of my own and I really wanted the freedom to make changes to my programs quickly, without having to consult anybody else," he says. Trent has developed the McEntire Workout Method and certifies successfully all over the United States. His growing network of supporters and activities surrounding Pilates include the creation of the "Pilates Challenge," a competitive event.

Of course, the bigger the endeavor, the more personality, endurance, and self-motivation become critical. We have to be outgoing and enthusiastic, and we have to really know what we are doing. A well-rounded certification program will greatly enhance our potential of making it through the first year. We have to be perfectly clear on our Pilates philosophy because this is the essence of what we are providing. Soloists are known to develop methods and equipment, and attract students because of what they have to offer. We may attempt to grow into a huge corporation, or we may stay small.

Often, trainers want to go solo because they have life experiences that make them experts for a certain population. The Center for Women's fitness in Ann Arbor, Michigan, for example, focuses on prenatal and postpartum courses, and the founder Carolyne Anthony developed a program on the ball after having three kids and little support from the fitness community. So she has ten years of experience, she has created videos and manuals, and she offers certification courses. She was even invited to teach her course at the last Mind Body Spirit conference and has been asked back. This has resulted in several people walking out of a conference with her certification program under their belts.

When you are on your own, expertise differentiates you from the average studio that will cater to a wide range of people. It is a performance, and you are the soloist, with all the responsibility that comes with it.

Still Unsure About Which Way Is Right for You?

In a gym, you wear sneakers. In a Pilates studio, you wear socks or are barefoot.

As a soloist, you can do whatever works.

In gyms, we have all sorts of tops, bottoms, jackets, sweat rings, towels, water bottles, sports bags, music machines, and vitamins. In a Pilates setting, we will put on a pajama-like workout pant with a little top, and off we go.

As a soloist, you can have your clients take their pants off when they slide on the Reformer doing stomach massage.

In gyms, clients are encouraged to buy fitness equipment for home use (athletic clubs are masters at point-of-sale revenue, and it means income for the trainers). In Pilates studios, trainers may start off by advising their clients to use a mat and practice their breathing until they deeply understand the principles: no money for equipment involved.

As a soloist, you will have to make decisions on what you really believe in and are therefore prepared to sell, and you have to be able to convince your clients through your workout that the item is useful for them. As a soloist, if your client's foam roller gets bumps and looks like the French Alps, on which it is impossible to balance (why do they always do that?), your client will bring it back to you. You had better give him or her a refund.

Fancy gyms often have juice bars, and people spend HOURS seeing and being seen. A Pilates studio will usually have a fast turnaround, with clients coming and leaving on the hour.

As a soloist, you have constant appointment changes. Clients call and you try to accommodate. It's called "personal service," and as a soloist you are likely to want to throw your phone in the bin many times.

In the gym, you have to have high energy and be outgoing all the time. In a Pilates studio, you need to be more "mellow," and even in a group class, competition is kept to a minimum.

As a soloist, you have to pick up the mood of your client and adjust your behavior accordingly. It is always about the client, never about you.

The Gym pushes you. A Pilates studio picks you up where you are right now. As a soloist, you are a hybrid between a marathon runner and sprinter. One requires endurance and careful movement, the other power and velocity.

Can you provide both?

The right place for you is wherever you feel most comfortable. If you are an energy bomb, like to show your body, are a great sales person, and love to learn many different fitness variants in a given year, the gym is right for you. If you like to work out in a communal setting, have body issues and a life story linked to Pilates, and want to work in a more relaxed atmosphere with feedback and support from other trainers, go for the Pilates studio. If you have many ideas and the zest to pursue them, are energetic and have people sensibility, go solo.

All of these options give Pilatistas a stage to perform that is in line with our philosophies and life experiences on a mental, emotional, and physical level. A work environment that reflects our philosophies will gain momentum almost by itself, it just feels so right.

Pilatistas are unique. I guess I will try and teach covered in leeches tomorrow and see if I can pull it off.

Maybe not.

3
Marketing
from the Core

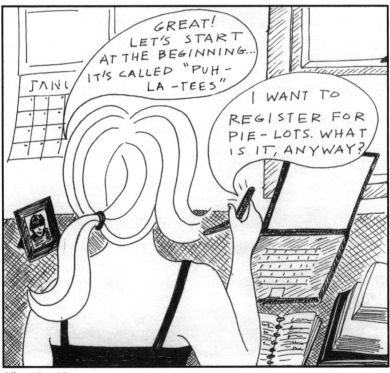

Off to a Good Start

We drive down the street, open a magazine, or log onto the Internet and are bombarded with advertisements. Advertising is everywhere. If done well, advertising creates interest and excitement; if done poorly, it can drive people away. In addition to referrals, marketing materials and Web sites are our main points of contact with new clients who are looking into Pilates. So, a little thinking about marketing is warranted in the mind-body community.

Holly Furgason, dancer, Pilates teacher, and designer extraordinaire, has worked with many Pilates teachers and movement professionals. Here are seven tips to help you enhance the representation of your work and make your business thrive!

Marketing from the Core

Holly Furgason, Interkinetic Creative Group

You have a great studio, but how do you get the word out? You know you need a logo, business cards, photography, flyers, posters, and a Web site, but where do you begin?

As movement people, we do not spend a lot of time writing. Many studio owners experience writer's block when it comes to sitting down and putting their thoughts on paper and presenting them to the outside world. Begin with your Pilates philosophy and write down some key elements with which your clients can identify.

I recently worked with a successful, experienced studio owner with a thriving business whose philosophy was not perfectly clear, and the conversation went something like this:

I asked, "What do you think will be on your Web site?" The studio owner answered, "Well, my logo..." And then there was silence. I had to start extracting information from her and use my best judgment to guess what her business was all about.

You know your business better than anyone else does, and therefore your active participation is fundamental to the design process.

Working with a designer is highly collaborative, and therefore, you should employ a designer who is interested in this line of work, who has an appreciation for movement, and with whom you feel comfortable. The graphic designer you retain should be seen as a creative resource; you don't have to know exactly what you want because he or she will guide you through the design process. That being said, a little preparation can save you money, increase your clientele, and enable you to present your business more professionally.

The idea of putting your business vision onto printed material and online can be intimidating, but it is by far one of the most important things you will do to launch your studio successfully. Here are seven basic marketing tools that a graphic designer can help you create and helpful tips to keep you moving in the right direction.

Marketing Tool 1: Logo

A logo should reaffirm your philosophy visually. You may have a very clear picture in your head for your business' logo, from the color and placement of the text to the details of the illustration. Alternatively, you may not have a single clue how to represent your business graphically. Both approaches are perfectly acceptable to any good graphic designer.

Depending on the amount of money you spend, the designer will produce one or more logo prototypes for you. Collectively, you and your designer will hone in the one design that best communicates your business philosophy. Make sure it is something you can live with—it follows your sense of style and business décor and you could see it printed on studio signage or merchandise such as T-shirts and water bottles.

What makes a good logo?

- It is immediately recognizable.

- It conveys the studio philosophy, ethos, and mission.

- It will look good small (1/2 inch) or very large (15 feet).

- It is timeless, not trendy (Will it look dated in five years?).

Tip: Collect ideas or examples of things you like. A page torn from a magazine, scribblings on a cocktail napkin, or a business card from a competitor can be creative inspiration to you and your designer. Place them in a folder, and take them to your design consultation.

Marketing Tool 2: Business Cards

Business cards may be your first contact with potential clients. Because of this, it might be worth spending a little extra money here to have top-notch, professional cards.

How can I save money on business cards?

- Stick with the standard size card (2 x 3.5 inches) and standard weight card stock, and use minimal color. Thicker, colored, or textured paper, printing on both sides, and multiple colors will cost a premium. Decide what is essential to the image you wish to present and what is just icing on the cake. If you are developing a newer studio, ask yourself what you can live without until the studio is fully established.

- If possible, print your cards in bulk. Most printers have price breaks when printing 500 or more at a time.

- Ask your designer to supply quotes from several printers so that you know you are getting the best price.

- Your local quick copy center may have business card services. You supply the logo and text, and they produce the layout and printing. This is a good way to produce cards quickly without having to pay for or commit to a large volume.

Tip: Once your business cards are printed, carry them with you in a cardholder, planner, or wallet pocket. Digging around in your bag only to pull out a worn card with bent corners is a poor representation of your business and a waste of the money spent to produce clean, crisp cards.

Marketing Tool 3: Photography for Print and the Web

Few things scream amateur louder than bad photography. Good photography takes time and practice. Start shooting everything! Over time you will have a significant number of quality photos at your disposal.

Before shooting, be sure to ask permission from your subjects, preferably in writing, to keep on file. It is not recommended to just take photos of a group class and post them on the studio's Web site. It is bad etiquette and could lead to a lawsuit. Typically, clients are willing, and even flattered, to be included, if they are asked first.

What will make my photos look more professional?

- If using a digital camera, capture the images at the highest resolution available.

- Scan the photos at a minimum of 300 dpi (dots per inch). This gives the designer more flexibility.

- Lighting is arguably more important than the camera itself. It doesn't make sense to use photos of poorly lit figures doing indeterminate exercises on marketing material.

- Simplify backgrounds by removing unnecessary objects that will just distract from the subject.

Tip: Find examples of photographs that you like in magazines or online, identify what it is you like about the images, and then try to recreate those aspects of the setting and lighting in your own studio.

Marketing Tool 4: Flyers

A flyer template is a must (usually 8.5" x 11"). With very little time, everything from special class offerings to studio announcements can be easily inserted into your template, posted, or emailed out. The easiest way to produce a professional yet flexible template is to have a designer produce a layout in a program you own, such as Microsoft Word or Microsoft Publisher, so that you can use it over and over again.

What makes a good basic flyer?

- Your logo and business name are clearly presented.

- The colors used will look good posted around your studio.

- It looks clean printed in black and white or in full color.

- It doesn't need to be cut or trimmed.

Tip: Is your flyer effective? Good design helps the reader's eyes navigate the page. Assessing the effectiveness of a flyer is easy! Stand several feet away from it, close your eyes for a few seconds, and then when you open your eyes, notice where your eyes go first. Hopefully, your focus will be drawn to the primary message of the flyer, which may be conveyed with text or with images.

Marketing Tool 5: Posters

Poster and flyers are different in scale and in use. A flyer is a more informal advertisement that typically is one page or a leaflet and is meant for wide distribution. Posters are large format announcements, usually 11" x 17" or larger. Movie posters are good examples of this type advertisement. Large format posters are costly but can be a very effective marketing tool. You want to design a poster that you can print in large quantities and distribute over time for special purposes.

How do I future-proof my posters?

- The information on your posters should not be liable to change. Really think about the essential content so you don't end up throwing them away after six months because the information is no longer applicable.

- Make sure your studio's name and contact information is prominently located.

Tip: Think about a poster as a way to advertise your studio in general more than a single event or technique.

Marketing Tool 6: Studio Schedules

Consider this: what is the point of having a schedule? Sounds like a no-brainer, but the answer is actually quite involved. A good schedule provides information about the times and types of classes being offered, entices clients to try something new or different, and subtly shows clients the studio's diverse and growing class offerings.

What makes an effective studio schedules?

- Be consistent with the look and layout.

- Make the schedule easy to navigate and understandable at a glance.

- Find a location in your studio and always have it stocked with the current schedule. Clients will get used to picking it up there.

Tip: You want busy clients to pick up the schedule and instantly think, "That fits my schedule," or "That class sounds interesting," without a lot of effort or interpretation.

Marketing Tool 7: Web Site

Retaining a designer to build the Web site is recommended in most cases. There are a lot of inexpensive computer programs that allow anyone to build Web sites, but good design involves much more than simply being able to put information on the Web.

What makes a good Web site?

- Content! It is surprising how many Web sites look amazing but don't provide any information or usable content.

- A Web site is useless if the information contained on it is outdated. Maintaining the site will only require a few hours every couple months depending on the size of your studio. If you intend to maintain the site yourself, make sure you indicate this to the designer at the first meeting as it may affect the software that the designer chooses to use.

- Navigation and the overall usability of the site is the key to helping viewers find information.

- Optimizing graphics, images, and special content for the Web is very important. If you do not do this, the Web site may load slowly or be sluggish to navigate. A potential client may become impatient and leave the site.

- Start with a basic site, and then add functions over time. You probably don't need an online store if you don't have any merchandise to sell yet.

How can I organize my thoughts?

- Prior to building a Web site, you must define the goals and objectives for the site. Some examples of objectives include recruiting new clients, creating a sense of studio community, and providing information or additional resources on techniques offered. Take the time to think about your Web site goals, and then clearly and concisely articulate them on paper.

- You must define your audience. Is this site for current clients, prospective clients, trainers, trainees, or some other audience group? Probably, it will be a mixture of all these groups, but depending on your goals, it may need to be weighted more heavily toward one group or another. Write down your audience groups and then rank them according to importance.

- Make a list of reasons why you think each audience group would be coming to your site. Make sure you address each of these needs.

Your Web site goals, the ranked list of audiences, and the list of reasons why various visitors would come to your site will be invaluable resources during all stages of the design build, they will help you and the designer stay on track, and they will ensure that you won't be disappointed with the end product.

Tip: Go online and find example of Web sites that you like in terms of overall look. Make a list of these sites and include simple comments stating what you like about each site.

Putting It All Together

This may sound like a real challenge, but when you work with a designer who understands your business, the synergy between ideas and skills will produce a product that you will love.

Final Tips:

- Graphic designers are expensive, but the beauty of Pilates is that you can trade almost any service for classes. If trading is out of the question, graphic designers' hourly fees are typically representative of their training, experience, and creativity, and, in most cases, the amount of effort they are willing to put into you and your project.

- Ask your designer for a thorough proposal that includes copyright details (do you own your logo or are you just "using" it), Web site maintenance costs and other fees associated with hosting, turn-around time for changes and updates, etc.

- Designers are not proofreaders. Make sure YOU see a proof of all printed material. It would be a disaster to print 500 business cards with the wrong address.

- Retain a CD Rom of all developed material and make duplicates of this CD. Having the materials in several formats will ensure your ability to use the logo over and over again for very diverse projects—from T-Shirts, bags, and bands to newsletters and posters.

- Templates simplify your work, reduce expenses, create a unified look, and make it easy for clients to surmise how important information will be conveyed. Templates for flyers and schedules are recommended.

- Ask permission to use any graphics or photos you find on the Internet, in books, or in magazines.

- Strive to be clear, clean, and simple. Design does not need to be complex to be effective and make an impact. Good design should inform and facilitate communication.

Marketing tools may seem to be somewhat cold and inhuman forms of communication. But in mind-body fitness marketing, you are "selling" something much more complex and important than a product—you are selling a person and a teacher who potential clients can trust with their bodies. You will know your design is right when it speaks to you—be clear about your philosophy and let it be your guide!

□ □ □

4
Anatomy Ready to Wear

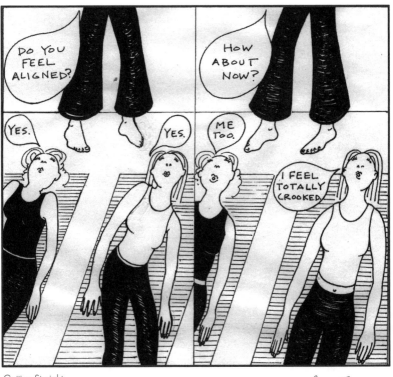

Getting Straight

t's Only Anatomy, and I Like It!

Anatomy is scary. Anatomy sounds difficult. Anatomy has a lot of strange, long, weird Latin names. Extensor digitorum longus pedis. Extensor digitorum longus pedis. Who can remember that?

Apparently, it all makes total sense if you have had years of Latin. "Extensor" means to extend, "digitorum" are the toes, "longus" means long, and "pedis" is the foot. So this guy is the long extensor muscle of the toes of the foot. Lovely. Scary.

When I started preparing for the Pilates exam, anatomy terrified me. "Somewhere in my leg," I answered when I was asked to locate my femur in our required 24-hour anatomy course.

Remember now, I am a dancer. I should know where my femur is. It is not exactly an entity as complex as the extensor digitorum longus pedis.

The femur is a huge bone in my leg.

Bottom line: I just wanted to die.

Muscle Hell

The muscles, their origins and insertions, and on occasion, their several heads, seemed to have a life of their own when I plunged into the matter and started to study viscously. I was determined to make all that Latin bone and muscle hell mine.

I was out of luck.

"Origin and insertions are old concepts that don't really apply anymore," a massage therapist who I was reviewing with told me.

Oh great, the one thing that I thought I understood, the "beginning and end of muscle," so to speak, was being taken away from me.

"Origin and insertion are dependent on which bony side is fixed," the therapist tells me. What does he mean, "bony side fixed"? Which side, what bone, and why fixed?

The flabbergasted look on my face prompted him to further venture into the secret realm of muscle workings: "The muscle levator scapula, for example, supposedly elevates the shoulder, according to its name. 'Levare' means to lift, like elevator; the scapula is the shoulder blade. There is a problem though. This muscle only works as an elevator of the shoulder blade if the scapula is mobile and the neck fixed."

Are you still with me? No? It gets worse.

"If you freeze the shoulder blade, this muscle will tilt the head sideways, toward the fixed shoulder. So in the first instance the neck is the origin and the shoulder the insertion. In the second instance it is reversed."

Aha. Ok I got it: A levator scapulae (elevator of the shoulder blade) can also be a depressor capitis lateralis (lateral depressor of the neck), right? It all depends on which bony end of the muscle is paralyzed for whatever reason. Five years down the road and many frozen shoulder blades later, I understand what he meant.

The Latin-speaking anatomists got it wrong. They had no time to reverse all the names, because they were forced to cut up cadavers in the middle of the night, risking their lives if they were caught. And now we suffer!

Pilates People

The people who choose to take on Pilates may have a strong exercise background, or they may not. They could be in such pain that you are stop number 456 on their path to recovery, or they may be striving to change their bodies to achieve a certain look and have heard that Pilates can do the "trick." Furthermore, clients come from different religious beliefs, are male or female, are with or without children, stem from cultures with differing views on touch, and range from overweight to underweight. They represent all racial shades of the human spectrum but, overwhelmingly, they are ADULTS.

We are, in fact, teaching adults who are beginners in the Pilates technique.

You may wonder why this apparently small piece of information on the makeup of our client populations is so critical. Why? Because our area, teaching adults, is one of the most neglected in the realm of learning research.

There are thousands of books on motor development for children and many more on how to teach children to move, but there are very few books addressing useful teaching techniques for adults.

Research on teaching movement to adults is geared toward the mentally or physically challenged. There is no funding for research that explores how we can teach adult novice ballet dancers to learn this technique more efficiently, although this population makes up a significant portion of dance schools. Likewise, there is no research on how to teach Pilates more efficiently, although some organizations are beginning to encourage the exploration of such topics.

With adults, it is crucial to teach skills that are functional, and can therefore be integrated into everyday life. Adults are busy and have families, partnerships, and a work life. Everything has a stake or value to it. Taking time to explain the value of the Pilates method therefore becomes important to fuel motivation and build a relationship, especially since the physical changes may take some time to manifest themselves. The client needs to have trust in us.

"How long will it take until I see results?" is a frequently asked question by new Pilates clients. "It works immediately, but it takes time to show," is what I usually answer. Joseph Pilates' promise that you will have a new body in thirty sessions is absolutely true, but nobody believes it.

The reason they don't believe it is that they assume that it relates to the body "look." What it relates to, however, is the mind-body connection. The value of this work, the value clients can store and retrieve any time, is the connection itself. These connections are the bridges that make change possible. In order to make connections, we need information. This enables the clients to envision how the puzzle of many elements that form the base of a good method comes together and relates to them. If Pilates exercises get them out of pain and they are able to pursue activities that they love again, such as skiing, golfing, dancing, or just walking, they will know that it works. Oftentimes they become even better at their preferred sports than before the injury, and they come to learn how to help themselves.

"My back is giving me problems today. Could we do the stretch on the barrel, then some bridging, and just work with the tennis balls for a while?" a client demanded when she walked in the other day. I was in heaven. Pilates a la carte! She was empowered and knew exactly what worked and what didn't. She connected the problem to a solution. The solution was specific Pilates exercises and stretches.

It is the connection that clients pay for. This is their investment.

Giving Value to Bodywork

If we buy an expensive piece of clothing, we get relief and comfort from the fact that we will be able to wear, display, and consequently store the item in our wardrobe for a long time. Dressy clothes are a good example of something that has a high price and low usage but becomes vested with value because we can store it.

How often do we really wear something very special and expensive? Seldom, but we keep it in the original package, neatly stored in the depths of our closet. Sometimes we may even take it out, not because we are going anywhere, but to feel the fabric, reassert the value of it (thus reducing guilt for buying something that we never wear but that was really expensive) and store it once again.

With bodywork, asserting value is complicated. Although the perception of wellbeing and feeling great is often immediate, we cannot store these feelings for a long time. If we only take one class, the feeling will gradually wear off. We are therefore asking clients to put time, money, and concentration into something that is not palpable at first.

Our society has a hard time investing money into something as unpredictable as our bodies. Doing Pilates is an investment that requires a relatively long time commitment, thought, and effort, without guarantees. Probably, a body will change significantly if the training is constant, but we cannot tell exactly how it is going to look. Taking the body alone for a gauge is an equation that will not work. We just cannot store sixty dollars worth of training in our bodies the way we could store sixty dollars worth of items in a box.

The mind, however, can store emotions, feelings, and information forever.

Magical Moments

"A good teacher should be able to create those magical moments, when the penny drops," say Lynne Robinson, director of Body Control Pilates in the UK. "The whole room is buzzing when you have made one person realize and discover something about their body and posture." Those moments make a difference for us, for the clients, for their bodies, and for our understanding of the relationship between these elements.

Pilates teachers use anatomical words to describing body parts all the time. Body parts are second nature to us and we are tested on our anatomical knowledge during the instructor training exams, so it can be tempting to flash those Latin words that took so long to memorize to our audience of clients. The Pilates "lingo" starts creeping into our teaching communication and confuses our clients. Claudiane Brum Vieira, a Pilates teacher from Brazil, told me that this had just happened to her. After three years of teaching someone, he looked up and said: "What exactly do you mean by neutral spine?" She could not believe it!

We assume that clients understand when we label bones or

muscles. Due to the inherent division of powers that characterizes the practitioner/client relationship, clients will often pretend to understand what we are saying. It is uncomfortable enough to join a movement class if you have never moved. Even worse is joining a movement class where the teachers asks you to locate your "TA" or engage the deep pelvic floor or nod from the base of the skull. Brent Anderson, put it this way: "We have no idea what a vertebra looks like to them." Let's make sure that they know what we mean. Dig out the bone man or the anatomy book; at least you will be on the same page.

I am adamant about the fact that we should teach basic anatomy to our clients. Our clients are adults; they can get it if we did, and they will progress faster and be more motivated if they understand what we are talking about. They will also be encouraged to look things up themselves and question more.

Does the teaching of anatomy need to be overly precise? No, it does not, but it should be close enough to provide a visual, verbal, and kinesthetic road map to the client's body.

Anatomy Ready to Wear

How can we go about teaching anatomy quickly, offering information about evolution and posture, and providing a direct application to the exercises?

Books are awkward to handle during a class and do not give a good visual representation of the layers of the different muscle groups. Using the anatomy coloring book, where you can learn about the human systems by coloring different layers muscles, bones, ligaments, and tendons, is very helpful but time consuming. Building muscles in clay is very informative but goes beyond the scope of a brief information session.

Anatomy is a huge block of information to master for aspiring teachers and clients alike. It is crucial, however, for making the right connections. I developed the following workshop according to three guidelines that I had set for myself:

1. The workshop could be covered in 5 minutes of class time.

2. The information would include visual, verbal, and kinaesthetic cues in order to involve everyone in class.

3. It should be fun, because positive emotions (and laughter qualifies as such) have the best chance of being remembered.

You will need the following items of clothing for every person in your class. If people are very shy and reserved, I show it all myself. Get ready to be laughed at!

You need:

*   A very small G-string (thong)

*   3 Dyna Bands in different colors

*   A flip chart or large self-stick Post-it

*   A marker

Stand up in front of the class. Introduce anatomy as a facet of the training and dive right into it. Climb into the G-string and if you have a relaxed class, ask everyone to do the same. The G-string will simulate the deep pelvic floor muscles. These are the muscles that everybody talks about, but nobody knows where they reside, what they do, and most interestingly, why on earth we should strengthen them. Write the name of each muscle group down on a flip chart, or write them on Post-its and stick them on the wall.

The Pelvic Floor

What are the two deep pelvic floor muscles called?

1. **Levator Ani muscles**

2. **Pyramidalis muscle**

The Pyramidalis muscle is, technically speaking, an abdominal muscle, but due to its location, it can be seen as a deep pelvic floor muscle.

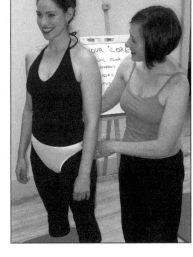

What do they look like?

The levator ani muscles are fan shaped, connecting the pubic bone to the tailbone.

The pyramidalis muscle is a triangle and lives on top of the pubic bone.

How do I feel them?

Squeeze and release the muscle which stops the urine flow. "Zip up your tight jeans" also seems to work well.

What do they do?

The levator ani muscles elevate (lift) the anus. They essentially control urinary and bowl movements and support the weight of our organs.

Why should we strengthen them?

The levator ani muscles are important for experiencing greater sexual pleasure and avoiding incontinence or a sinking of the bladder or womb.

The pyramidalis muscle assists in thoracic flexion and pelvic floor contraction.

This much will make your clients remember where the pelvic floor is—forever! There is a lot more to this interesting part of our anatomy, if you care to read on.

How We Lost Our Tails

The deep pelvic floor used to be a prime device for communication. This was in the days when our semi-human predecessors had not yet decided that standing up was such a good idea. When we spent most of our time as quadrupeds on all fours, the deep pelvic floor was still controlling bladder and bowel movements, but on top of that, it was responsible for emotional communication.

An animal's tail tells it all! Tail moving = come along, tail down = I am sad, tail up = get off!

With humans standing up, there were physical adjustments to be made. The stomach was relieved of its mule-like, organ-supporting job, and became a weaker area of the human structure because it was left with no gravity-related purpose. As a result, our back muscles also suffered (more about this later.)

The deep pelvic floor, however, had to become very strong to take over the task of carrying our organs, and our tails curled under to create a platform for these new heavy-duty muscle actions.

This development took away our tails. I am mad about that, because it seems like we have lost a great way of telling people if we like them or not. Maybe I would not write a book on communication if we had kept our mood-signalling, personal traffic light: the tail.

Try to discover the reduced signalling actions of the tail(bone). Think a happy thought. What happens to the body, can you feel it lifting and the tailbone extending, therefore releasing backwards? If we had a tail, it would raise like the tail of a happy cat or dog. Then try the reverse. Think about something that saddens you. Notice that hunched shoulders will make the tail curl under. "He has his tail between his legs" is not just a saying, but a physical reaction to an emotional state.

Today, we are making another shift. Since we decided to spend our time balancing on our sit bones all day long, the deep pelvic floor is having major problems in our era of computers, desk jobs, and sedentary life. We sit while doing countless activities that required activity for the past generations: driving instead of walking, sitting at the computer, paying our bills online, drive-through restaurants and ATM's—it surprising that we still are able to walk at all!

In a sitting position, the deep pelvic floor is stretched out. When we walk, especially when swinging our hips, the deep pelvic floor works. Unfortunately, even when we walk, swinging our hips is considered inappropriate. Again our pelvic floor is asleep.

Let's look at another, perhaps more disturbing, example. Women gave birth squatting for thousands of years as opposed to lying in a hospital bed, on their backs, with the tailbone blocking the birth canal. "In this position, the baby has to literally bash under and around the bone to come out." Carolyne Anthony told her petrified class in the prenatal Pilates course.

Why are women still lying on their backs to give birth? Good question, but be prepared for a terrible answer.

Because the supine position is the most comfortable for the DOCTORS.

Knowing that, we have just found one of the most compelling reasons for teaching Pilates to gynaecologists. For a woman-friendly delivery, all mothers-to-be need is a strong core (in order to keep their upper body flexion for hours), plus good lateral rotation. Criss-cross is the perfect exercise for the woman-friendly gynaecologist!

If there is a performer in you, this history section calls for physical enactments! We are not just teachers—we are entertainers as well! Have your clients walk on all fours. Tell them to lie on their backs imagining the tailbone closing the birth canal passage and ask them to give birth.

What a huge amount of information, anchored to a small G-string! Be warned, this part of the session takes longest, because people are usually in stitches by now.

Now we can proceed to discover the other layers of our abdominal muscles.

Sing It! Serenade the TA Muscle

Write the name Transversus Abdominus down on the either your flip-

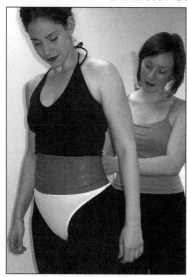

chart or Post-its. Next, grab one of the Dyna Bands, and wrap it tightly around your waist. Have everyone do this one with you. Make sure that the lower part of your transversus abdominis muscle attaches at the top of the G-string triangle.

What is the deepest abdominal muscle called?

Transversus abdominis. Transverse means across, and the abdominis is the abdomen.

What does it look like?

This muscle runs across the body (transversally) and wraps around the waist like a belt.

How do I feel it?

Sneeze, cough, or laugh holding your hands on your waist. Sing a note for as long as you have air.

What do they do?

The transversus supports our back, makes us laugh and cough, and helps during flexion and extension.

Why should we strengthen them?

The transversus is our most important back support muscle. It divides and creates space between our hips and our ribs, thus decompressing pressure on our digestive organs.

The TA muscle is the deepest of the abdominal muscles. It hugs us tightly and is responsible for contractions such as laughter, cough, and short, pressed sounds, such as the ones you hear when a martial artists hits something (Huagh!). It is also crucial to have a strong TA during pregnancy in order to have the strength to push the baby out. We need a strong core to push. Pushing works a lot better with sound, which is one of the reasons why I found that singing during Pilates classes is great for activation of the abdominals. Although there is no research to support this, I also find that people with scoliosis are able to recruit both sides of their abdominals a lot more evenly when they sing during a roll up. All of a sudden, they do not compensate toward their stronger side as much.

Using sounds to find the TA muscle is an easy way to increase awareness and explain the potential of the muscle. Have your clients stand up, take a deep inhale and sing the "A" sound for a slow count of ten. Due to flat breathing habits and a weak TA muscle, the first time around, your new Pilates crowd will probably only be able to hold the sound until the count of four or so.

Depending on the size of our lungs and the power of the TA muscle, we can sing a note and hold it for a very long time, as long as the breath flows slowly and constantly. The TA muscle will press out the air and create a girdle around us. We can apply sounds to every exercise in the Pilates repertoire. It works beautifully in extensions, when clients tend to use their necks to get extension or during the roll over, when a lack of thoracic flexion will create strain on the cervical spine. If the breath cannot flow, the spine is not aligned, and we will get a constricted sound. The sound then acts to reinforce the correct movement.

Use this exercise as a gauge for your clients' improvement. After ten weeks, singing and counting to ten will be easy, and feeling the TA will become second nature.

These exercises are also very compelling visually, since the band will loosen as you activate the TA muscle on the exhale. Needless to say, a slim waist is a good by-product of a healthy TA.

The most important element in this round of anatomy, however, is the fact that the TA attaches to the spine, it supports the back. "You need strong abdominal muscles to take care of your back pain" may make sense to a PT, but for clients who know little anatomy, it does not.

We need to make clients aware that the Pilates method works because it makes sense, on many levels. Teaching anatomy is one of them.

The Obliques

Now the second Dyna Band is ready for action. Use it like a shawl, passing it around the back, under the armpits and down to the pubic

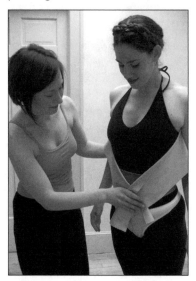

bone. In the front, the muscle looks like a "V" and inserts into the top of the pubic bone. Make a small knot and let it rest on top of the pubic bone.

What is this layer of abdominal muscles called?

Musculus obliquus, which means muscles that run diagonally.

What do they look like?

They wrap around the lower part of the ribs, in a diagonal, "V" shape.

How do I feel them?

You can feel them during rotation, making the ahh sound, and in flexion.

What do they do?

They assist in flexing the torso and are responsible for rotation of the upper body when the pelvis is fixed.

Why should we strengthen them?

The obliques support the back in extension and rotation.

For the sake of time and simplicity, I visually treat them as one muscle, omitting the internal and external fibres of these trunk rotators. Although by omitting the internal (hands in pocket) and external (hands away from pocket) fibres of this muscle, we are not technically 100% correct, we can give a good visual, sensory, and verbal idea of this large muscle group to our clients. Exploring questions such as: "How do they move with exhalation? Do they work synergistically with the TA? Do they support the back?" Make it easy to find the answers. Yes. Yes. Yes.

Now the message is loud and clear. Strong abdominal muscles can relieve back pain because they act as stabilizers and balancers to the whole skeletal system.

Undoing the Six-Pack Myth: Rectus Abdominis

What is this layer of abdominals called?

Rectus Abdominis; Rectus means straight, and the abdominis is the abdomen.

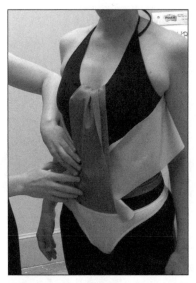

What does it look like?

This muscle is thin and long, and is divided into four compartments on each side. The muscle starts at the front of the breastbone and runs down into the pubic bone.

How do I feel it?

Flex your torso and push the stomach out.

What does it do?

The rectus helps with flexion but does not support the back. It is often overworked and can be prone to diastatsis, a splitting of the muscle.

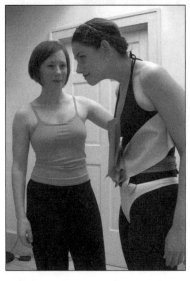

Why should we strengthen them?

We should not strengthen the rectus on its own. A tight rectus pulls the upper body into a curve.

This is my favorite part of the anatomy session: to enlighten my class about the famous six-pack muscle and reshape its myth of power and beauty.

1. It is not a six pack but an eight pack. Two packs are hiding in the Pyramid muscle.

2. It is the only abdominal muscle that does not attach to the back; it therefore does not do anything for your back issues.

Having said that, a strong rectus abdomini muscle does something. It will make us lose a few inches in height if trained accordingly and give us a nice, forwardly rounded, upper-body curve.

When you demonstrate this, take the Dyna Band and stick it into the top of the client's shirt (close to the breast bone) and then let it hang down loose. In order to simulate the over-trained Rectus, put the band into the G-string and pull tight downward. Since the head will naturally follow the path of the spine, the client is now kyphotic. Needing to see where we are going calls for an adjustment of the neck. It now extends in turtle fashion. Looking good!

Voilà! Your client is cured from the six-pack myth.

Common Ground

Humor aside, this anatomy lesson combines research for successful learning and retaining approaches as found in the scientific literature. Using all our senses and asking questions are the most effective ways to teach and the best ways to learn.

We have just done it all as suggested in the literature: we used mixed modalities of teaching. We used patterning, metaphors, analogies, role-playing, visuals, and movement in addition to reading and writing. We have been able to feel the shape, size, and action of each muscle. After the ready-to-wear anatomy session, you will have a whole new army of Pilates supporters who will go out into the world and talk about muscles and posture endlessly to their friends. And, they have not even done a single exercise yet!

We have created common ground. Your clients and you are now on the same page—they know which words you will use, they will have experienced flexion and extension, they can now attempt the exercises with understanding and feeling.

The gates for building a mind-body connection are now open because your group speaks the same language. Change happens a lot faster when we have reasons why we do the things we do.

It is the mind that will motivate us to practice a movement over and over in our own time, using imagery, recalling touch, and remembering verbal cues. Independent clients will soon help themselves and keep coming back for more connections. The possibilities for growth are infinite.

Anatomy is a scary place no more!

5

Fit to Teach? Do Logokinesis.

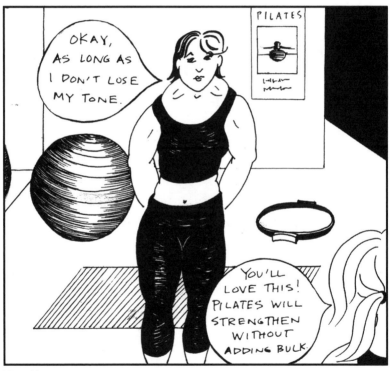

Mirror, Mirror. . .

will never forget when a well-known teacher came to Rome, Italy to teach. The class was scheduled for 1PM on August 5th.

Clearly, a non-Italian had to have set up this schedule! Air conditioning is not a given in Italy by any stretch of the imagination. In August at 1PM, 99% of the population is having a siesta with all their windows closed to keep out the sun.

In this instance, the timing of the workshop could have had two potentially negative results. Either nobody would have signed up for the course and our teaching talents would have never gotten a chance to surface, or the heat at that time of the day would have made movement impossible and teaching ineffective.

Environment is only one of the peripheral areas that heavily influence our clients' ability to understand and ultimately transfer information into long-term memory. There are others as well, and it is useful for our teaching practices to keep them in mind when we greet our clients and organize our studios.

From a wealth of studies on learning and memory, it seems clear that our clients learn best when we follow these three guidelines:

1. Acknowledge clients' emotional state.

A quick "how are you?" asked with interest and intent goes a long way here to give you an idea of what has happened in the day of your client so far. Remember or review your notes of your last conversation with her. Was an event coming up? Was she having discomfort? Was there a new exercise you introduced that worked quite well or not at all? How did she feel after the session? What are her goals for this session?

Listen for the tone of your client's voice, as Elizabeth Larkam suggests. Is there tension? Does he speak really, really fast; can you already tell that it will take a long time to get him "down to earth"? How are you going to accomplish this? Or let's look at the opposite scenario:

is the client moving slowly and looking like the weight of the world is resting on his shoulders?

Moira Merrithew, co-founder of Stott Pilates, suggests asking for the client's motivation and goals when they take up Pilates. "We should avoid dictating to a client what their needs are," Moira points out. "We can notice things, such as their posture and energy, and utilize exercises that will address those issues, but we should respect their needs and speak to them about their goals."

Once we have acknowledged the spoken and unspoken things about a client, we can devise a strategy, or plan a journey, on how to best serve him or her. What follows are my personal suggestions for approaching this.

In my experience, a busybody—a person who has high energy, runs all day, is on the phone constantly, and has a really hard time focusing on anything—can be brought down quickly by getting his or her heart rate up right at the beginning of the session.

The hundreds are a good exercise here, or sometimes I also crank up the music and have client bounce on the ball for 10 minutes to Earth, Wind & Fire's song "September." (People LOVE bouncing on the ball to music. I think there is a really deep, "back to childhood" element in this simple exercise. I have a blast doing it too, of course.) After this intermezzo, they can go back to breathing principles and calmer, more concentrated activities. This kind of approach also works when people are angry, because any type of cardiovascular activity will release endorphins, the so-called happiness hormones.

The low-energy clients are different. We need to take them to a better place through the workout. I usually start with the principles and choose exercises that they are good at. Being positive is really important; they may also be very much up for touch and assisted stretches. We give our energy to them through touch.

Many of us Pilates teachers come from a dance, fitness, or other movement background. This can create a false assumption that the population at large is comfortable with and adept at perceiving their bodies. Our motor skills are very refined when we compare them to those of the normal population, who sometimes have trouble performing basic movements, such as activating an arm in conjunction with the opposite leg.

"Do not assume anything. Ask," Alan Herdman, a revered British Pilates practitioner, points out.

Asking about the daily physical state of the body is good and warranted. The body is different every day, but sometimes we do not pay attention to it. Questions such as "How are you?" or "How is your body today?" will initially be met with suspicion by the new Pilatista. "Nothing. I'm fine," will be a common reaction at the beginning. Listen to your client's answers. If everything seems to be fine, that's a warning sign. Keep going with your "cross-examination."

"What about your feet, legs, hips? Has your lower back being troubling you? Have you been sitting a lot this week? How are your neck and shoulders?" It may not seem like much, but we are actually teaching them about feeling their bodies.

The most amusing thing that happened to me recently dealt with exactly this issue. I was teaching a new Pilates mat class in a dance studio. I asked about injuries. Everybody was "fine." When I started the class I noticed that one participant had very unique body patterns. After twenty minutes, she said: "I cannot believe I forgot to tell you this, but my spine is fused from the lower cervical to the mid-lumbar spine." What?! How could she forget to tell me even after being prompted?

People get used to their bodies and may be unaware of them, so asking persistently is a good way to go!

Number two in order of importance in learning relates to physicality.

2. Meet clients' physical needs.

When our clients come to see us, they could have been running around for too long without drink or food. They may have been affected by the cold or heat outside. They may have disorders such as diabetes that heavily impact the way they can move. A teacher from the Australian Pilates Association told me that she measures a particular client's sugar level when he comes to the studio. She always has nuts, dried fruit, or a power bar available—and if one day his level is just too low, she sends him home. That's the real meaning of caring about clients on many levels!

We should also have water or herbal teas in the studio and encourage clients to drink during the session.

Once a client lies down on the mat, any thought regarding physical needs (this includes the trip to the bathroom) should have been met and be out of his or her mind.

Finally, let's look at the studio environment.

3. Provide an environment that is inductive to relaxation and concentration.

This section refers to the studio itself. Are the spotlights shining into your client's eyes like a hot iron rod when they lie on the mat? That is not relaxing.

Is it freezing cold or too hot? They will not remember a thing you say and be very uncomfortable. Last winter, there was a problem with the heater in the studio where I was teaching. You could literally see your breath in the morning. Those were clearly not the best classes I ever taught; I should have cancelled instead.

Is the music too loud, the teacher next door too vocal? Attention is diverted even when small things are perceived as invasive.

What about cleanliness? Are the mats or the equipment covered in dandruff from the previous client? (Yuck!)

People notice, and we had better believe it will make a difference. Attention is key to a successful studio.

Once we have paved the way for our clients to give us their undivided attention, the next big milestone to effective teaching is communication.

In the old days, people thought that the best way to teach was to inflict some sort of intense emotion on their students; hence they came up with physical punishment. Way back then, and in some countries to this day, teachers say something and if the student doesn't get it or fails to pay attention, spanking is on its way. That will work! Or so they thought.

In this century, neurological research showed us clearly that the whole learning experience is not all that straightforward after all. There is no question that emotionality paired with information does make us alert. After all, if someone holds a knife to my throat, I will certainly pay attention and see what the person wants from me.

What researchers found out though, is that punishment only makes us do what the perpetrator wants from us as long as he is right there. We do not internalize that information as something meaningful for us and will therefore stop our pleasing behavior the minute we feel free! What makes things meaningful to us is positive feedback and common goal setting. Communication theories today take into account that the only way to teach effectively is to be highly interactive with our students. We must ask questions, define goals, and assess performance for good results.

This is the theory. As with all theories, it misses the human component. That's why I came up with the concept of Logokinesis. Logokinesis encourages you to do some spring cleaning and reorganize your closet of life experiences related to teaching so that others can benefit.

Logokinesis: What's in the Word?

The Greek word "logos" means "word," "argument," or "ways of thinking." "Kinesis" comes from the Greek word "Kineein" that means "to move." Basically, I am encouraging you to take anything that interests you, makes sense to you, inspires you, and moves you and integrate it into your teachings of movement.

My interest lies in communication, so I experiment with different approaches to teaching, such as a communication model called neurolinguistic programming (NLP), and try to integrate them in my classes. You may be interested in neurobiology or music and use your beliefs in that area to make your teaching unique.

It does not matter what the interest is—what matters is the wealth of experience that your clients can gain from it.

Before we start with the ins and outs of this teaching model, Kim Dunleavy, a physical therapist at Wayne State University and doctoral candidate in teaching technologies, mentioned a key fact: "The mind can only focus on a small number of elements at any given time, typically 7, plus or minus 2," says Kim. "When we start teaching a novice learner, we may be tempted to give too much information. The client goes into overload and the information itself becomes an element of distraction."

Of course, that's the last thing we want. So we need to give limited, focused bits of instruction. Here is an example, instead of saying "Stretch your leg," during single leg work on the Reformer, it is more helpful to say "Stretch your right leg." This directs the client to the leg we want to see stretched.

Another absolute "no-no" is something in which we all like to indulge. Don't say "don't."

Why? Because it requires your poor clients to do double the work. If we say "Don't tense your shoulders," our clients first visualize tensed shoulders and then have to undo that image and work backward. We are providing negative reinforcement (what we don't want) instead of focusing on positive reinforcement (what we DO want). "Relax your shoulders!" would be the effective way to cue tensed shoulders.

Imagine a stop sign that reads, "Don't Keep Going." It would take us several seconds longer to realize that we must stop than if there were a simple "Stop" sign. Now that you are aware of it, you just might cringe every time someone says don't!

Kim also thinks that it is important to differentiate novice learners from experienced movers and adapt our feedback accordingly. A novice leaner does better with feedback that describes how a movement should look, rather than focusing on how it should not look.

An experienced mover, however, who is used to corrections, can do well with visualizations of the wrong way along with suggestions on how to fix it.

Suggestions for fixing things will make us tap into the realm of learning modalities. We all learn differently: some people are more auditory learners—they like lots of information and information delivered at a fast pace. Then you have the visual people, who learn best with images, or the kinesthetic learners, who react to touch or to phrases that evoke feelings of pressure, texture, and intensity. In a mat class, it is pretty much a given that all types of learners are represented, so we should make sure that we include elements from all of those areas in our teaching.

Alastair Greetham, a physical therapist with an interest in neurolinguistic programming (NLP), did a great communication workshop at the last Polestar conference. He had us write down cues for the three different modalities. I had the hardest time coming up with cues relating to images; that is my weak point. Get a piece of paper and write down cues you normally use. Are they more visual, auditory, or kinesthetic? Then go ahead and try to expand your vocabulary in the areas that seem underrepresented. These will need some practice!

Motivation and goal setting are very important, as mentioned earlier. When introducing a new exercise, there are several things to consider.

Phase A: Teaching a New Exercise

Stage I. Introducing a New Exercise

First we must formulate the objective of the exercise. Single Leg Stretch, for example, could have two different lines of focus.

We could choose to focus on core control, keeping the knee at a 90° angle and therefore increasing the leverage on the abdominal muscles;

Or

a. We could focus on hip flexor and hamstring stretch, prompting the client to take the bent knee in all the way into the chest and reaching the extending leg long.

These are essentially two different exercises. Good programming requires us to make a decision and formulate an argument behind it. This way we teach our clients the following:

a. Pilates exercises can be modified in essence and scope.

b. Essence and scope are personalized to the needs of the client.

c. As long as the principles are observed, there is not really a right or wrong way to do an exercise; it depends on the objective

These three elements combined basically make up a good method: a good method is all-embracing, meaning that the principles can be applied easily to any type of movement; it is also flexible in orientation, meaning that it can be modified to fit our needs.

Objectives are a road map for your clients. Your clients know exactly what they are supposed to work for that day and can respond to it. Objectives are also important for us as teachers because they make programming more consistent and make us think about modifications. It is helpful for our clients if we stick with a theme once we have settled on it. If we have stipulated the objective for the class as being on shoulder girdle stabilization, it is very frustrating and unfair to the client to shift focus right in the middle of the exercise. It reminds me of dance classes, when your teacher told you to be more expressive and dance more and then, when you were on verge of letting go, she zoomed in on a not perfectly stretched toe.

"Complexities are an amalgamation of short simplicities," as New York City Ballet principal Edward Vilella said in his master class. We need to deconstruct movement until the body is able to move on to another task level.

Stage II: Modeling the Exercise

Clients need to see the end product of what they are supposed to perform. Showing them an exercise the first time we introduce it is only fair. The objective is to give a blueprint of the movement and then move on to the next stage.

Stage III: Client Performs the Exercise

Start by setting up the exercise slowly. Name the exercise and the objective again. "Now we are starting Single Leg Stretch, focusing on or abdominal muscles, therefore only bending the knee at a 90° angle." Take it slowly, cue the breathing. Have them say words out loud as they move through the exercise. I frequently have clients or a whole mat class say the words "up" or "reach" when they perform movements in upper body flexion. The result is amazing: the body curve remains the same or even increases, therefore summoning up more core strength. Best of all, the information sticks.

Words are the gateway to our thoughts and help us master a movement.

Words are prime motivators. When you think about extreme situations that you need to get through, what is it that keeps you going? I would argue that it is self-talk. Steve Madrid, a seasoned marathon runner, reports that self-talk carries him through the run.

Self-talk, or encouraging yourself that you can do it, will help you do it! It has amazing powers when used along with movement.

Stage IV: Seek Feedback

Ask your clients how the exercise felt. Could they reach the objective, did they feel what you intended for them to feel? Prompt them to talk about more things that related to the exercise. Did the breathing pattern feel right? Was the speed good? Did the self-talk make their effort more intense?

If you are satisfied with the response, let that exercise go and move on to something familiar. If not, repeat it and seek feedback again.

This type of approach actively involves your clients and empowers them to accept responsibility for their own bodies and health. Increased knowledge creates more interest and will encourage them to do things at home. People LOVE knowing things about THEIR bodies and posture, and ways to improve them. This is what they should get when they invest in personal training—a personal, unique, informative, transforming experience. You can bet that when practicing at home, self-talk is the one element they will readily use when gathering motivation.

Phase B: Reinforcing the Information

I mentioned before that the Logokinesis approach happens in different stages. We had four stages to our introductory exercise session (Phase A). The second, reinforcing session is crucial to the anchoring of kinesthetic information.

Stage V: Client formulates the exercise

As soon as your client comes in and has settled down with a gentle warm up exercise, you can pick up the discussion about the new exercise you taught him or her. Prompt your client with questions. What was the name of the exercise? What were its goals? How did it feel?

Stage VI: Client teaches the Exercise

This part they love, because they get to teach YOU! Build in some mistakes as they guide you through the exercise. See how they correct you. This will give you important clues on how they learn. One of my mat class clients had to teach the Hundreds once. He blew us away with a blues, finger-snapping, foot-tapping rendition of the breathing. It was great. If we think about it, you can only teach someone else well if you know what you are doing. Using this approach, you teach your clients what it is all about.

Stage VII: Client Performs the Exercise

Now we are back on the mat, and the exercise is done by the client. If you like, you could also add a modification at this point.

Stage VIII: Joint Feedback and Playtime

Quickly check in with your client's perceptions. Did your client meet the objectives? Does he or she have any comments? How difficult does he or she rate the exercise? Play with possible modifications or your client them to come up with an exercise for the next class.

Anchors for Wellbeing

Accepting the fact that people come to us with a busy schedule behind and in front of them calls for some tricks of the trade in order to help them get comfortable quickly. An hour is not very long if it is takes us 20 minutes to relax a stressed client or comfort a worried one. The notion of anchors comes from NLP. Basically, it involves using a stimulus (in this case, a scent) to reinforce and anchor a movement or state of relaxation in a client. Anchors are bridges that help you transfer from one state to the next with ease. The two anchors presented here are aromatherapy and alignment through touch.

The Oil Bar

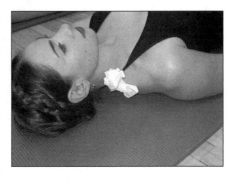

The oil bar at the studio has been a great success since I first started using essential oils as a means to anchor and relax clients who had a hard time concentrating when they came into the studio from the "outside" world. We carry a selection of six oils (mandarin, lavender, peppermint, eucalyptus, rose, and lemon) with descriptions of their qualities on a chart. Clients pick the oil that best reflects their mood on a given day and put one drop on a Kleenex tissue. The tissue is then placed in the back of their shirts or is just tucked under the top end of the mat. The scent immediately fosters concentration and relaxation and is a wonderful "entrance" to the breathing principle of Pilates exercises. In this case, aromatherapy also functions as an anchor to the studio. Since there is no direct contact with the skin, allergic reactions are avoided. As with all oils, get a book to educate yourself about those populations who should use scents with care, such as pregnant women.

This practice is common with massage therapists, who use eucalyptus oil placed on a tissue under the headrest. There are two advantages here! For one thing, the clients' noses don't run and drip on the floor, and for another, this particular oil provides decongestant and antiseptic qualities. In the winter, when clients have colds, using eucalyptus oil is great because it makes them feel better and it helps us to be less prone to catching the flu.

Glenda Taylor describes the powers of aromatherapy in her book *Aromatherapy: For Relaxation, Beauty, and Good Health.* Scents can conjure up associations. If these are pleasant, the body is more prone to activate self-healing powers and indulge in the feeling of wellbeing.

Smells also make you look forward to something. Try this! Close your eyes and think of your favorite meal, one of those that a special person has to make, otherwise it doesn't taste the same. . .I can, right this moment, smell the aroma of my mother's lemon butter cake, even though she lives 6000 miles away and there is not a cake in sight in my house.

Scents become an anchor for wellbeing, which is in turn associated with Pilates, the studio, and the instructor.

Alignment and Massage

Touch is a luxury these days. We are not a very physical society in terms of showing our affection to people outside of our partnerships and families. If you have small children, you are lucky to enjoy millions of heartfelt kisses per day, with no restriction, no backward thoughts, just pure and simple love.

As a Pilates student, I was always drawn to teachers who have the gift of touch, and it has somehow carried over into my classes. When a client first lies down, take a moment to look at him or her. Your hands will be drawn automatically to a tension spot or to a misalignment. Gently stretching the neck or helping to release the shoulders or the hip joint with small movements creates closeness and is often appreciated. It also provides you with a muscular road map of a body. It is hard to explain, but I usually need to feel the texture of the muscle before I feel comfortable devising exercises. I really like to assist clients while they exercise or stretch. There is such a wealth of feedback in touch.

If we jump start an exercise without realignment, we probably zoom right into our tension spots.

"First realign, then exercise," says Carolyne Anthony, director of the Center for Women's Fitness. "Through gentle manual realignment, you reprogram the body to neutral, and the breathing will do the rest!"

This is why I never skip the warm-up portion of a Pilates class: the breathing, the rib cage placement, the connection into my body is by no means given when I sail into my class from the outside world.

Using touch during teaching is a problematic area in our community. Some states specifically forbid touch unless you are a certified manual therapist. Still, many of us use common sense and intuition when making the decision to use touch or not. Elizabeth Larkam says: "I determine what is appropriate. I can certainly cue a whole session without touch, if I feel that the client feels most comfortable with this approach. We should ask and be gentle."

In German we call this approach "Fingerspitzengefühl." Directly translated, it means "Finger-tip-feeling." We need to tune our conscious and subconscious receptors to the needs of the person in front of us. I have yet to meet someone who has not welcomed the "gift" of touch. Just be aware that if you do not feel comfortable touching, there is no rule saying that you have to. Sometimes it feels more awkward to touch someone we do not want to touch, than to avoid touching that person altogether. Do what feels good to you and the client.

Teaching Movement is a Living process

Planning gives confidence to your clients and encourages them to trust you. We do not want to promise benefits that are unreasonable, such as loosing weight very quickly or transforming a normal body into Elle McPherson's.

What we can promise are the rewards of consistency. The so-called "hopeless cases" never fail to amaze us when they finally make an active decision for change. Humans have unlimited capacity for reinvention. As trainers, we will never be able to do it for them, but we are the anchor for a good starting point.

Essentially, teaching is a communal activity, a living process. Through learning, we establish communion and can therefore hope to achieve transformation. Alistair Greetham gave us one really good piece of advice at the end of his communication workshop: "This is powerful stuff. We should always use communication skills with good intent and not as a way to manipulate people."

When language, information, and touch blend perfectly in your classes, you will be on top of the world. Your clients will take the information and run with it. You will have the power to reinvent yourself and what you teach constantly, becoming an endless source of creativity. You will be a joy to be around, and people will gravitate toward you naturally.

"Work" rarely gets better than this!

6

Your Client and You:
The Therapeutic Relationship

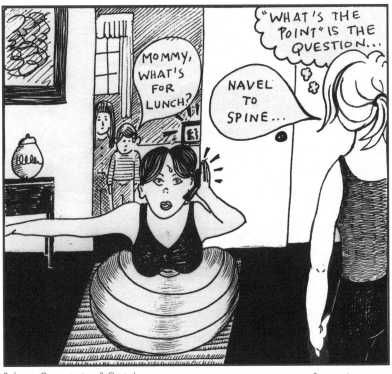

Balance, Concentration, & Control

D o you see the comic at the beginning of this chapter? The lady on the ball talking on the phone? The children "interrupting" the session asking for food? The TV going full blast—and me in the middle trying to teach?

Well, this is only half the picture. There was no space left to add the violin practice of one of the kids, the landline phone ringing every ten minutes (it has a beautiful balletic ring to it: tam, tam; tam, tam; like a preparation before pliés at the barre), and my client talking, not in English, but in Spanish, while bouncing on the ball!

I love this family and have known them for years.

The scenario described above is only one of many that make up the so-called therapeutic relationship. The therapeutic alliance is a rational agreement between client and practitioner in which the parties essentially agree on a "contract" which will support a goal or treatment. The alliance at its most basic could be a patient with a physical problem who visits a doctor qualified for the type of problem that the patient is experiencing, and the client placing trust in the doctor's ability to diagnose. The doctor then will investigate, make a diagnosis, and prescribe a treatment, assuming that the patient will comply with the recommendations made.

This sounds pretty straightforward when we are dealing with a scenario such as: "I have a cold," followed by, "Yes you have a cold, I will prescribe you some medicine for it." In a training scenario, expectations and needs of the client are usually a lot more complex. The complexity of our relationships with clients combined with a lack of training on how to handle those cases with which feel uncomfortable, is the focus of this chapter.

It is a chapter about client assessment, professional integrity, and boundaries. It is also about topics that were alien to me before researching for this book, such as transference and countertransference in the client-practitioner relationship.

Choosing our Work Environment

Feeling professional is to some extent related to our environment. If the above description of a Pilates session is totally alien to you or you think that such "working conditions" are not acceptable, I hope you will read on. The way we feel about working environments is people related. If I am treated with respect, if my work is valued, if I feel like my time means something to my client, then there is no problem. As long as respect is intact, we can decide to be professional in any environment. My point is that we could work out of the most beautiful space in the world, but teach awful clients who are racist or sexist or think that we are some dumb trainer who does a "low-level" job. Would we put up with it, just because of the exteriors?

The other aspect to consider when setting up working rules is the population we teach. A prime example is mothers of very young children.

Oftentimes, mothers will call our studio and ask for home sessions because they do not want to leave their newborn babies. Carolyne Anthony, whose main interest lies in teaching pregnant and postpartum women, loves having them bring in their babies to the studio. She is perfectly happy carrying most of the babies on her lap in turn, cueing exercises while entertaining the newborns.

In her arms, they smile and sleep. In my arms, however, the opposite occurs. Ten minutes into the postnatal class that I was subbing for, ALL the babies were crying. (This also happened on another occasion, when I did a lot of shoulder girdle work with them. I did not know that the gland that is responsible for milk production sits right below the scapula. . .ahem.)

When we make choices about our environments, we can do whatever feels good. For Carolyne, this class scenario is perfect. I felt totally overwhelmed.

Assessing Our Clients

Clients have different personalities and we who are training them will require a certain amount of "people" skills to be effective. We cannot have a special relationship with everybody, nor do our clients demand it.

Eric Franklin talked to me about this at a conference. "Responsibility from a teacher's perspective requires him or her to acknowledge the mental, physical, bio-mechanical, and emotional elements that make up the human in front of us," Eric says, "but also asks of the teacher to establish boundaries that will enable him or her to keep working with many people daily without feeling drained, and possibly becoming ill."

"It is important to realize that whilst you can not help everyone, you should have good will and interest to refer your clients to other practitioners if necessary." Eric continues, "The difficult thing in assessing a client is recognizing that there are several key elements that make up human beings."

According to Eric, we can use the following structure to assess a client:

Mental Element: We should look out for reoccurring thought patterns that seem to characterize the mental state of our clients. Are they mostly positive and open for suggestions, or do they criticize everything and everyone and seem to have a rather gloomy outlook? Are they energetic, or do they qualify as "energy suckers," making you feel like you just taught five hours in a row instead of one? Assessing the mental element can give us a good indication on how to handle their comments, without taking them too personally.

Emotional Element: This may be more difficult to spot in the beginning. Feelings of anger or guilt, for example, have deep repercussions on our bodies. Eventually, after a while people will make side comments that relates to feelings of anger or guilt if they have them.

Physical Element: What kind of life activities do they pursue? Their jobs and hobbies may involve a lot of repetitive movement that will affect their readiness to be physical. If someone has not moved for years, their body may have limited resources available to do a full workout, and we need to program accordingly.

Biomechanical Element: This refers to overall skeletal, muscular, and organic state of our clients. We are usually well-trained to assess the first two elements, but may have little information about organs. Look at their complexion, hair, nails, and teeth. Ask about nutrition habits and check if they drink enough water or consume sugar-loaded sodas. Check about their digestive systems: constipation has hardening effect on the whole core and oftentimes those problems get a lot better quickly once you start making them breathe and work through their spines.

After this initial assessment, we should ask ourselves, "Can I really help?" We need to watch out for altruistic patterns. In this profession, we all have them to some extent. Once we have decided that a particular therapeutic alliance is going to work, we really get to know not just the client, but the person. I asked several instructor teachers how they suggest we handle clients who can be a little more "problematic." The following common issues came up:

The Talker

The talkers, or Pilates "Alibists," are those clients who use their Pilates session as an "alibi" since they would much rather be social than work out! These clients know that fitness is important for their health and they want to look good, but generally speaking, they cherish the social component of fitness. They are also usually very interesting to talk to, which makes it harder to avoid being sucked up in conversations with them. So, what should we do if two-thirds of the class is spent talking?

This is a sensitive issue. Eva Powers, Master Trainer for Stott Pilates and a Professor of Dance at Wayne State University, has years of experience mentoring trainers of all ages. Working in a busy studio, she has had the chance to study client/trainer relationships on a daily basis.

Eva's approach is clear and has integrity: "If clients want to talk, it is the trainer's responsibility to keep them moving. Unfortunately, it is often the less experienced trainers who indulge in the chit chat and seem to have a hard time getting the client to focus. When I ask them about it, they tell me that the client is happy and has the right to use their time however they wish. Our reputations, however, suffer from this. It is always better to be known as a focused trainer, who challenges the client appropriately every time, than a 'talker.' The clients will complain eventually because we have not provided the service that they paid for. Needless to say, the physical results will not happen either."

Personally, I would suggest that one reason that younger trainers feel less confident to direct clients who talk a lot is age difference. I feel weird interrupting people who are older than I am. Usually, I just listen and do a lot of back extensions when possible. It is a lot harder for clients to keep talking when they are lying on their stomach as opposed to on their backs.

Eva has the perfect solution: "Work them out a little harder; they will thank you in the end!"

The "I Don't Feel Anything" Client

Another type of client is the one who has low or nonexistent body awareness. Even identifying different body parts is difficult for these clients, and they seem to rarely think about how their bodies feel. This is especially prevalent in older individuals who have never exercised before and are starting with Pilates late in life. They may have completely missed establishing neurological pathways that allow them to recruit and access different muscle groups. This can be very disconcerting for the trainer, who is lost for ideas on how to make it happen. These types of clients have a greater chance to develop body awareness through the resistance of the equipment. A mat workout will probably not be sufficient to achieve substantial change to keep your client motivated. Using equipment for feedback can do wonders for them!

This of course is diametrically juxtaposed with our own body awareness. The more attuned we get, the fewer "perfect days" there are. My business partner Aimee and I joke about this a lot. A frequent conversation goes like this: "How are you?" Answer: "Oh horrible day today. The lower fibers of my left QL are tight!" And off we go to try to stretch out.

The Client in Pain

Clients in chronic pain go through waves. Their tendencies to look for the reasons for the pain will increase on a bad day. (Was it sitting in the car? A bad pillow? Vacuuming?) A lot of times, I have really been frustrated with myself when I think the client may be able to try something else slightly different, and his or her body reacts immediately. Seeing a client walking out of the door in worse shape than when he or she walked in is really terrible. However, we can only assist the client to the best of our ability and take it one day at a time. I would suggest that small doses of Pilates several times a week instead of one full hour per session is best for this population. Sometimes though, things can also change for the better.

Clients with chronic pain will praise Pilates to no end once their pain has subsided. We are happy, they are happy, and things are looking up. Interestingly, very soon, the pain is forgotten and an unrealistic perception of abilities starts to set in. All of a sudden they want to enjoy their newly found pain-free state by exercising harder. It always amazes that when I work with a person with terrible back pain and disc problems for six months: we get it under control and before you know it, they decide to run a marathon, bike some mountain, or go ice skating!

I also love the shift from "pain management" to "cosmetic management." There is no talk about back pain, but lots of talk about the shape of their legs, tone of arms, and in-depth analysis of other body parts. Witnessing this kind of journey is one of the most fulfilling aspects of teaching Pilates.

What If a Client Gets Hurt in Class?

I spoke to Nancy Hodari of Equilibrium Fitness about this. Injuries can happen even to people that appear to be really strong and ready for a new exercise. Sometimes old injuries flare up, other times we may have misjudged their abilities. Other times still, a new position that they have not been in before makes them tense up and they forget all the principles in a heartbeat. The exercise becomes "dangerous." Nancy suggests keeping meticulous notes about every session. As a lawyer, she knows that in court, only good note keeping makes a case for the teacher. Did the client mention a new source of pain in the previous class? Was there any unusual activity in the class? Write down the programming so you can make a case for consistency of training. As for her own experience, Nancy says that, "overall, in the years the studio has been running, there have been only minor incidents. The clients have been great. One lady who hurt her wrist kept coming with her arm in a cast."

Regardless, we don't have any way of predicting what could happen if one of our clients is injured. We should make sure to buy insurance! Both the Pilates Method Alliance and NAMASTA offer this through their Web sites (in the US only). In order to protect ourselves as trainers, client-practitioner boundaries should be understood and made clear in our interactions with our clients.

Boundaries

Boundaries are frames of action in which both the clients and we feel safe. In order to feel safe, we need to know where we stand, and this is true for any aspect of a relationship. By being clear and honest, and working with good intent, we establish good boundaries within which we can safely navigate. The three most commonly described boundary issues of Pilates teachers were issues of friendship with clients, money matters, and working out good trade agreements. Let's go through them one by one.

Client Friendship

We care deeply about our clients. We worry about them and they worry about us. In the last years, there has been more than one terrible scare, because one of my clients got cancer, another was getting divorced, another had trouble with her kids, and others still suddenly lost their jobs. How can we witness all of this and not be involved? Do we not become "friends" in some way?

It's not all gloomy either: there is also joy about births, weddings, and communions, and uncertainties when somebody applies for a new job. Some people leave town and say goodbye. The last time it was me who left and relocated. My clients in Hamburg, however, are still in my heart. I know what they are doing, if they are well, if their partnerships are okay. In a way, I think we grow with every relationship, and the client relationship is no exception.

We are to some extent involved with our clients' lives, especially those who we have known for years and really like. We may get invited to parties and functions. We sometimes talk to them on the phone about things other than training. We ask for help. In a small community especially, converging interests such as art or dance create social interaction that goes beyond the boundary of a Pilates session. Potentially, crossing over from professional to social can be problematic. In reality it is often unavoidable and I would not want to miss it.

Most of our clients are referrals. Our clients therefore know each other, talk about each other and (sometimes) talk about us to each other. They know when we are back from a trip even before we have had time to make one phone call. They sometimes even switch appointments. Last week, there I was expecting person A but person B shows up. Best of all, they promote us and our work and they love us!!

There is a downside to this, however. Knowing and teaching a group of people who know each other brings up issues of confidentiality. Clients sometimes tell us their secrets and even if they don't, their bodies can give us a good indication of their mental states. Confidentiality in the therapeutic relationship should be handled much like the attorney/client and doctor/client conduct. We should not share confidential information with anyone else even if they appear to have been told much the same thing. We simply don't know what they consider private and what they do not. Our job is to make them and their information safe. Besides, we are on the hot seat. One small shift in an established friendship circle, one misunderstanding, and we are cooked!

Which other methods are available to keep confidentiality if the shared information really got to us? In Nina McIntosh's book, it is suggested that regularly talking about these issues with a mentor or supervisor greatly reduces the tendency to "gossip" about clients with other clients or other practitioners. This is a great way to "share the burden" and get advice from another trusted person who is a body worker as well. Psychotherapists and psychologists are required to have mentors; it would be just too much to cope with otherwise. Why not take their advice and get things off our chests so we are ready for our clients again? It's like cleaning out your hard drive.

Money

Juggling the dual challenge of being caring and an instrument for better health on one hand and accepting payment in return for a humanistic service on the other, is hard to do for many of us who are not able to stay assertive and separate the two issues. How do we feel treating, caring for, and healing a person and then, an hour later saying: "Gimme sixty bucks." It's weird.

Money matters include the basic pricing for the service we provide, but they also include whatever rules we have set up in case someone needs to cancel a class or reschedule, or if they drop out of a course altogether and want a refund. We need to have clear communication about our policies. Put up sign; have your clients read and sign a form contract when you take them on.

Money is not just a finance entity. Eric Franklin shared his thoughts on money matters. "Money is often mistaken for worthiness." Eric says, "you always have to balance the following power problem: on the one hand people want the 'best' of anything, on the other, they also want a good deal. Let me tell you a story of a massage therapist friend of mine. He had too many clients so he decided to double his fee in order to reduce the clientele. What actually happened was quite the contrary. Word of mouth that he is so good because he is so expensive went around really fast and he had more clients than before. Scarcity and elevated price creates more demand.

"Money is also energy," Eric continues, "Finding the optimal balance between power and energy is a psychological factor."

Money equals safety. Money is a boundary. It forces us to provide what our job description says that we will provide: training according to the Pilates method.

If we would advertise all over town that we teach for free (assuming someone comes), people will think that something is not quite right. They will be weary of what it is you claim to be doing. Since I started thinking about money as a form of safety, lots of things changed for me. I learned it the hard way. If somebody was not able to pay my rate but wanted training, I was likely to let the "little helper" syndrome take over. In my last studio, I taught lots of really nice people for less money than my regular fee. They referred more really nice people who could not pay the rate. Before I knew it, I was swamped with great clients who could not pay my original rate. I was working around the clock and getting exhausted.

No more. I gear my charitable actions away from the workplace and back to where they belong. Today I chose to donate work hours for non-profit organizations, but I keep these activities separate from my work.

The second part of money management, and the one I would argue we struggle the most with, is cancellation policies. In other words, what is our time worth if we did not work at all? Unless a client walks in and hands us the check out of his or her own accord, we have a really hard time enforcing our cancellation and payment policies. For me, asking is worse that not getting paid.

Moira Merrithew made me feel much better when I asked her how she dealt with money issues. "I must say that Lindsay [Moira's husband and CEO of Stott Pilates] has helped a lot with this, because I am not so good with money issues myself. Teachers need to be paid because they are providing a service, because they make a living with teaching and have to pay the rent."

Bless her! We are not alone in this! "Generally speaking, a 24-hour cancellation notice is the norm," Moira says. "This is 24 hours from the time of the appointment, not the evening or the night before."

There seems to be great consensus and agreement on the fact that money, cancellation, and late payment issues are REAL and EVERYDAY problems. "You can't win on that one," says Lindsay Merrithew. "We just have to deal with it the best we can!"

I collected a short list of "good things to say" when we are faced with an angry client who does not want to pay the cancellation fee or thinks he or she can schedule, cancel, and reschedule with joy and utmost non-sensitivity:

1. "As you know, I do charge for missed appointments."

2. "This time, I understand your situation and am willing to make an exception. Next time, please be aware that I will charge the full fee for a missed appointment."

3. "I only see a limited number of clients per week in order to give you the full attention you deserve. I cannot keep up my practice without a cancellation policy. I hope you understand."

4. "Everybody is happy here! We have never had anyone complain about this before! Besides, you signed the policy so I assume

you were aware of it." (This is my all-time favorite as suggested by Nancy Hodari, lawyer, studio owner, and baby boomer extraordinaire! It takes the ball out of our court and throws it back to the client!)"

Trading

Money is also not always measured with physical currency. I trade Pilates lessons for tons of things, and it has been problematic in some cases. In others, it was a wonderful experience. Trading is great, but we need some basic communication about the value, the hourly input, and the suggested end-of-trade agreement. Are we trading by the hour or by value? I would suggest that trading things that people make (such as clothes, jewelry, Web site, etc) is more difficult to barter against Pilates sessions because their hours may fluctuate. Therefore, we should agree clearly on how many hours of our services get bartered for exactly what kind of product. It is also important to clarify when the agreement ends.

I traded sessions for a pair of handmade, beautiful shoes for my husband's birthday. The shoes took three months to make, but due to schedule conflicts I was there paying them off with sessions for almost a year. Such a long-term trade does not work well for the party providing the service.

Even if the people we trade with are friends, sit down and scribble something on a piece of paper. Trades usually go to the bottom of the list of people's priorities. If you trade something as important as a massage and don't want to get bumped into crazy days and crazy hours, it may be well worth paying for them, call the shots in terms of scheduling, and enjoy it more.

As you can see from the above, guidelines for handling the therapeutic relationship exist. Did I know about them during my training or did anybody prepare me for these decisions? No.

Did I make many mistakes, some of them painful? Yes. Am I still encountering odd situations that call for sensitive decision making that has no "how to react" manual? Yes again. For these reasons, I think it would be useful to alert future teachers to these job-related occurrences.

It would be useful because knowledge gives us the tools to be alert and watch out for "red flags." We are talking about relationships. Relationships take time to build, but they also take time to degrade. Trust, sympathy, and special personalities can confound our judgment. On top of that, every client comes to us with a past. This includes childhood experiences as well as interactions with people who bear some of our same traits. At the other end, there are the practitioners, with our own pasts and traits. All the client profiles and habits discussed before are within the normal realm of things. We all have our ways, quirks, and habits. Sometimes, we can also encounter people with more severe problems, and we may get wrapped up in situations that we are not trained to handle.

Welcome to the world of transference and countertransference in the therapeutic alliance.

Transference

Transference is the unconscious projection of previous experiences to the present. Research in attachment theory (which is the study of how we form and maintain intimate relationships) has largely proven that the nature of our relationships is heavily influenced by our childhoods and especially by our relationships with our parents. So basically, our behavior is influenced by our perception of reality, which includes expectations, knowledge, and the attempt to be objective and logical, together with associations of our past relationships.

Transference is unconscious and present in any relationship. It is also important to note that although transference is something that happens, it is not necessarily bad.

In athletic training, for example, we often see transference in a mentoring relationship. A student is in awe of his coach because he needs a father figure and admires the coach's skill. Or, a student can not stand his coach because his autocratic training approach evokes bad memories he has of his father. This situation will go on for a while until the student matures and moves on. Feelings of transference can be positive or negative, but as long as the common goal can still be achieved, there is no need to address them.

Some personalities, however, are more prone to transference, and those are the ones that we need to watch out for. There are three different possibilities here, all of which should be considered red flags!

1. Rigid Personalities

These are clients who are very rigid in their thought patterns and possibly not able to reflect upon their wishes and problems actively. These people will project past experiences directly to your present relationship: they are too friendly one day and hostile the next. But they keep coming back to you regardless.

2. Vulnerable Personalities

People who are injured, sick, or find themselves in a very unstable domestic or social situation are also prone to projecting feelings and expectations that are outside of the ordinary "client/trainer" relationship. A sick or injured client, for example, who is scared and lacks confidence, suddenly assumes a childlike role with her Pilates teacher. The sessions are spent discussing her illness and her feelings of anxiety rather than doing what we are meant to be doing, which is practicing Pilates.

3. "Too Much" Personalities

Frequent contact is another indicator for increased potential of transference symptoms. As nice as it is to have a client who wants to train every day, there is enormous responsibility that comes with that. Who do we see every day? Our co-workers, spouses, and children. None of these people pay us; we are with them because we work side by side or because we love them. "Too Much" personalities are kind and loving people who have limited genuine social interactions and are in great need of love and attention. Imagine if a client were to start calling you twenty, thirty times per day, inviting you to dinner, and showering you with expensive gifts. We can easily get sucked into a weird drama of feeling responsible on one hand and feeling not completely genuine on the other. If we see a client every day, he or she could easily make up a third of our income. How can we remain objective in such a situation? I would suggest avoiding this type of situation by establishing firm boundaries. We can tell the client that three times per week is all that our schedule allows.

The literature suggests that cutting down meeting times may make the transference more complicated, like taking something away and triggering a "wanting more" reaction. It is important to honor the scheduled meetings in order to provide a safe framework for the client. Keeping our phones off and not answering messages in the evening or at week-ends is also a good idea in order to keep boundaries. If somebody seems to display "Too Much" personality profiles, just be firm and friendly. He or she is likely to direct the focus of his or her attention to someone else after a while.

As my partner Aimee McDonald put it in summing up her experience with a "Too Much" client: "She wanted my life and was mad when I would not give it to her."

Aimee made a really good point when she said that part of the reason that clients with this type of personality become so obsessive about their teacher, doctor, or aesthetician is because body workers are, generally speaking, pretty mellow and have made active decisions about what to do with their lives. "Too Much" personalities are also really likeable and have wonderful, caring sides to them. It's just all a little too much, and our lives can be greatly affected due to our reactions to this kind of transference.

Countertransference

Countertransference refers to the practitioner's reaction to of the client's transference. If we assume and act upon the role of the father figure coach and exploit that relationship, or if we play the "best friend" game with the anxious or sick client, we are caught up in countertransference.

It is difficult to spot countertransference if the responses solicited by our clients are in line with our normal personality profiles. If we have feelings toward a client that are in the normal range of our usual emotions, there is no need to worry. It is when we start making exceptions, bending the rules, or thinking about a particular client all the time (this can include sexual feelings and is one of the reasons why practitioners and patients should not cross that boundary) that we can assume that countertransference is happening.

Examples of countertransference include being angry because a client clearly insists on "not getting better." They keep coming to class and tell us that Pilates does not work. We may get frustrated and even angry, and either multiply our efforts (thus encouraging more adamancy about it not working from the client) or feel attacked and withdraw.

Feelings of love and attention are the hardest to be objective about. After all, who doesn't like to be wanted and loved?

Dealing with it all!

What helps me in knowing about transference and countertransference is that I can keep more distance and check my reactions objectively. When I see a new client, I do make a point of finding out about his or her natural state and make a mental note of it. Rigid personalities that have significant mood swings with no clear reason that we can identify, just need to be treated kindly and consistently kindly. We have to avoid reacting or wondering what we may have done wrong or nursing aggressions towards them.

"Vulnerable" personalities (sick, injured, or anxious clients) require careful monitoring of our comments and advice, since they are likely to ponder it and possibly misinterpret our good intentions.

"Too Much" personalities are actually easy to spot; they will flood us with attention and if we are alert about this, we can establish boundaries quickly and effectively. In fact, the following guidelines by Patricia Hughes and Ian Kerr at St. George's Mental Health Trust were very useful to me, so I will pass them along:

- We should question our behavior, attitudes, and motives.

- We must realize that we too have "soft spots" for people.

- We are affected by our clients and they are affected by us.

- Clients often have strong feelings toward us.

As a final thought, I think that in our profession, which is far less extreme that what is experienced by a psychotherapist or psychologist, the eventuality of such encounters is slim. We have a disadvantage, however: we are not trained to spot others or ourselves for issues of transference and countertransference, hence our chances of doing it all wrong with a handful of "problem" people over a Pilates career is very large indeed.

This quote by Lynne Robinson beautifully sums up how I feel about the overwhelming majority of my clients: fortunate!

"I feel that we are privileged to be in people's lives, that they share life with us. You learn as you go, life is a roller coaster. In a way, go you through divorce, illness, birth, marriage several times per year. It's an honor—we are very fortunate—but it does come with responsibility."

Choose your clients wisely. I am happier teaching people with a hectic life, including dogs, cats, parrots, and vacations, than being thrown into a relationship that requires different skills that the ones I have been trained in. After all, we teach Pilates, not psychotherapy.

7

Love, Sex, and Friendship

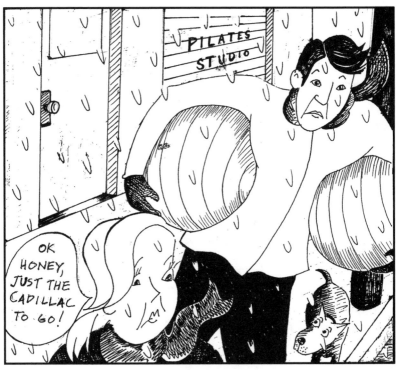

What I Do For Love

"I cannot even remember the last time I had sex on a Wednesday night," says Dana, an attractive, physically fit, 35-year-old. "I see twelve clients that day."

There it is, spelled out in black and white.

Now what?

I decided that writing about the issue of low sex drive in mind-body professions is important. It is important because many of us think that teaching Pilates is a healthy job. It focuses on relaxation, breathing, and body awareness. We preach about a balanced body that is influenced by and relies on a healthy lifestyle.

Why then, did every female teacher who I approached with regard to low sex drive reply emphatically: "Oh my God, I thought it was only me!"

It is not only us Pilates trainers. Low sex drive affects as many as 40 million women, according to a University of Michigan Health System press release. The most common non-medical reasons for low sex drive are stress, fear, and anxiety.

STRESS! The "no-no" word in the world of Pilates.

OTHER people are stressed, the ones who run all day, take airplanes, talk on the phone, and have to meet deadlines and make sales targets. We wanted a job that didn't require these stressful things.

There is no stress in our studios. We do not encourage competition or any other anxiety-inducing practices in our teachings. I would argue that we are certainly not allowed to show stress when we teach. Who wants to pay for that when they get it for free all day long?

So, what went wrong?

Nothing went wrong at all. We are not weird because we cannot make it all happen despite our being Pilates teachers. "What do you mean you are stressed?" one of my friends said when I dared to complain in a quiet moment, "you teach Pilates." She was really surprised, as if Pilates could make us immune to all the other worldly happenings to which we are exposed. As if working in the mind-body community exempts us from even being able to say that we are tired and, yes, stressed!

If there is a secret tool in Pilates to escape and transcend our daily lives, I have not yet mastered it. And I thought I was advanced. . .

We need to realize and accept the fact that we share the same world as every other man and woman who is working, raising a family, taking care of the house and animals, and has no time to him or herself. And if there is no house, husband or wife, or kids, the picture does not change enough to lessen much of the stress. Anxiety comes into play. We fear making ends meet, fear becoming sick or injured. Stress, anxiety, and fear are companions for many of us. Really, we are no different from our non-Pilates-teaching neighbors or friends.

"It is not just that being a Pilates teacher sucks your energy," says Nancy Hodari. "Being a working woman today in any profession sucks your energy, because women just never feel DONE with work."

If we don't have a family and dislike the idea of buying into the "I am stressed" theory, there is another avenue of thought in explaining low sex drive.

Partners in Life

"I have no desire for intimacy when I am working full time in the studio," a young female British Pilates teacher told me. "When I am on vacation, though, I really long for sex and my husband thinks I am going nuts."

This topic has been researched in the literature. The groundbreaking book for dancers, *Competing with the Sylph: The Quest for the Perfect Dance Body* by Lawrence Vincent, reported the next to nonexistent sexual activity of ballet dancers during a performance season, followed by sexual overdrive during their holiday period.

For athletes or dancers then, the high physical activity demanded from their profession pushes sex off the radar screen. When they are on vacation, however, and do not move at all, the body goes into movement withdrawal shock and needs to "exercise." Now sex comes into play again!

There is a problem with this argument in relationship to us Pilates teachers. We are not athletes. Even if we manage to work out an hour a day, which is almost impossible to achieve for many full-time teachers, we do not spend the rest of the day moving. We talk about movement.

Either way, the only way out is to balance our teaching schedules so that we have energy left for those who mean the world to us. If we constantly overexert ourselves, by the time we get home to our loved ones, they become another to-do list item. In the business of caring for others, caring loses its unique property of being something special you share with few people.

There's No Time

I can hear some of you already.

Nice thought lady, but what about the dogs, cats, kids, kids' friends, house, cars, shopping, and teaching? And what about money? And what about the pride I take in running my own business, being successful at it even though, oftentimes, the people I do it for don't appreciate my efforts?

Here is the account of someone who finally made a decision. "Gail" left her hectic life, her house, her husband, and her cats, packed up her three kids, and left America to teach in another studio thousands of miles away. She remembers the times before her decision to leave.

"On" All the Time

"Gail Teal," a Pilates teacher whose husband wanted her to stay anonymous

Sometimes it is hard to switch into my teaching mode in the morning after having spent three hours making breakfasts and lunches, doing two loads of laundry, feeding the cats, making beds, getting myself showered and dressed, and finally taking everyone to school. That's when I feel I need to have some time out. I feel I have already done a full day's work. Instead, I gear myself up for my clients.

I have already listened to my own family moan and groan, and now I put up my "The doctor is in" sign. Part of being a trainer is to also be a confidant. You have to try and balance the workout with a therapy session. Pilates has the tendency to release not just muscles but tongues as well. After teaching back to back for a couple of hours, I inevitably get a call from one of my daughters. This could be because someone is sick, has forgotten homework, is setting up a play date, or, most often, I have forgotten to sign a permission slip. It is off to the school to rectify these problems on my next break, which happens to be my lunch break. Lucky, I always have a Luna bar with me.

Since the school is also near the grocery store, I run in to get a few things for dinner. I never do big shopping anymore. There never is time. Then back to the studio/office to work.

My studio is in my house. I used to think this was great. Now as I put the clothes in the dryer and clean up cat vomit I realize: 1. I never go anywhere. 2. I am always doing something.

I work on the computer for a while before the next client shows up. Then it's off to pick the kids up.

Meanwhile, my eldest girl has got a lift home and has arrived with at least five friends. The house fills up as my second eldest girl gets off the bus with two friends and the youngest, who I have just picked up, has one friend in tow.

You count—how many kids in my house? AND THEY ARE ALL HUNGRY!

So off I go downstairs to teach another client. The noise level upstairs resembles a pop concert. After the fourth time running up and telling them to be quiet, I am working, I get mad and throw everyone out. "Geez Mrs. Teal, you could have told us to be quiet," is the response I get.

Finish that client and up the stairs to start dinner—which has to be cooked before the evening class at six.

Downstairs to teach—put up with the noise of family eating and watching TV. They have been told that I have a client, but because I teach at home it is not considered serious.

Two classes later and I crawl upstairs to have something to eat.

Then I clean up, put another load of laundry in the machine, feed those damn cats, check my email and the kids' homework, make food for lunches the next day, and make sure that everyone who doesn't belong to me has gone home.

Bed for me is at 9:30. I can't function after this—I get up at 5AM.

Some days my husband comes home late and wants to talk about his day. Never mind that I am asleep. SOME DAYS HE EVEN WANTS SEX!!! What is he thinking! I have noting left to give.

Weekends fare no better. I teach only on Saturday mornings. My kids think nothing of shouting down the stairs asking for soccer shoes or swimming suits when I am in the middle of a session. I do not exist as a separate person. Even my husband will mow the lawn outside the studio. Can you hear me? He asks incredulously when I complain.

After I finish teaching it seems to be a free for all—the kids come swooping down the stairs with friends in tow and start bouncing on the balls and climbing on machines.

Are they allowed? No. But do you think it makes any difference?

The only respect I get is from my clients who thankfully keep coming.

But things have to change, and the first will be a studio downtown preferably with a phone number that is not accessible to my family.

☐ ☐ ☐

The author of this paragraph has decided to come back from her 8-month hiatus to a far-away land. Her job was not what she expected, her kids missed home, and her husband missed all of them terribly. So, they are coming back to the United States after a huge learning curve for herself, her husband, and her children. Happier? Certainly. Wiser? Absolutely. Any regrets? Not at all. Sometimes you have to do what you have to do to realize that you like it at home the best!

But there is still the sex issue. Even if we reduce our teaching and have more energy for our partnership, there is a tiny, issue that's hard to get rid of. It's called routine: that daily, uneventful, emotion killer. Here is the rescue plan for our sex lives.

Sex-Rehabilitation-for-Body-Workers Rescue Plan

Any kind of sexual withdrawal/overload roller coaster is hard to integrate into a partnership. One of the byproducts of my interviewing Pilates teachers all over the world is that I came across issues of interest that I had thought about before, but never in conjunction with other trainers. I thought that my being tired all the time was my problem in my relationship. After all, spending hours talking nonstop and touching bodies all day long kind of makes us want to get away from it all.

In fact, isn't it amusing to consider that we talk about the pelvic floor as much as a porn star is required to talk about sex in interviews? Who on earth talks about something so seldom-mentioned and "private" as the importance of having a strong pelvic floor to anyone who walks into the door, male or female, several hours per day? This occupational theme kind of demystifies the whole pleasurable aspect of sex, don't you think?

"I spend so much time, frequently with men, discussing the deep pelvic floor on a professional level, that I got very good at wearing this shield," was another memorable comment from Elizabeth Larkam. "I had to work on enjoying movement as an avenue of pleasure, instead of analyzing it from a teaching perspective. Today I think that being the recipient of touch balances your input and output. To move and to be touched is such a fulfilling experience."

This is not to imply that we all have sex concentrating on the eccentric action of our pubococcygeal muscle, but maybe sometimes that happens too! People working a normal job do not spend that much time analyzing the formations and deficits of their sexual organs. For them, movement is seen as something they do in they spare time and for pleasure. It is a hobby, a way to detach and regenerate.

We, however, not only talk about movement and the body constantly, but have visuals as well. We look at people's bodies from the weirdest angels. How about the fine view we get when we cue leg circles on the reformer, observing from the side of the foot bar? Sometimes I think we get to know other people's deep pelvic floors better than our own.

When I think of a vagina, romantic pictures such as prolapsed bladder, incontinence, and other conditions come to my mind. "Penis" does not fare much better: prostate troubles, more incontinence thoughts, along with wondering whether men can Kegel or not are common thoughts that I court. Sexy, hm?

All of this is bad enough, you may think, so what else is there? The worst is yet to come. The worst part about this, dear fellow teachers, is that our clients report an ENHANCED SEX LIFE after they start Pilates.

Great! Lovely! Good for them! Meanwhile we get stuck in the Wednesday blues.

Unfortunately, this is not just our problem. We could just go to sleep and forget about it. The problem is that others suffer from this. What about the people carrying the burden of being married or partners to us?

A friend from England, married to a Pilates teacher, sighs: "All your friends think that because you are married to a dancer and Pilates teacher you are the lucky one. Great body, super flexibility. 'Mate, you got lucky!' Well, let me tell you, it ain't necessarily so. They are tired, they are exhausted, they don't want to talk when they get home, let alone have sex. They are Pilates mummies."

Maybe if we started to think about sex like bodywork, this would help. Maybe things would be easier if we started thinking about intimate touch differently. In fact, it would probably help if we would stop and think about intimate touch for a while, about the closeness, safety, and beauty of it.

Accepting this time as a time to let things happen is key: not being in control, not having to cue anything, just floating along. This would make sex feel like a place to reenergize, instead of becoming another energy sucker. Once we experience sex as being relaxing and energizing again, we will be more likely to be open and giving about it.

Schedule Change, Now!

We have to make some schedule adjustments if we want this to work. Teaching late every night of the week is a killer. The toughest element of working when others have time off is that we never have time off when others are working. We cannot join into the communal rejoicing of "It's the weekend!" exuberance. For many of us, the weekend and evenings are the money-making, existence-guaranteeing times.

We need time out from that. "Make sure you take a weekend off now and again," says Lynne Robinson, founder of Body Control Pilates. "Teachers need to go back into the real world sometimes. It's not good to live in the Pilates bubble. We must have a life, friends, and interests that are outside our work."

Sometimes we just need a little time to make the transition. Getting out of the studio early, having a meal with your partner, and putting some distance between work and personal life is helpful.

How can we go about this?

We need a bedroom facelift. Although this takes some orchestration first, it is fun and relaxing, and it will get your creative spirits going again.

Why the Bedroom?

Most people make love in their beds. Is this a fair assumption? Research on family communication seems to say so. Once the first period of getting to know your partner has worn off (and with it the love making in obscure locations, at unbelievable times with peculiar props), we stall: welcome home love routine!

The bedroom is such a terrible place for intimacy that I seriously considered separate bedrooms when I got married. The arguments were just so overwhelmingly contra-bedroom. How do I know? I researched family communication and sex. And I found out that the bedroom is a total turn off, not just for sex, but for good communication as well. A bedroom has the following characteristics, which are counterproductive for relaxed lovemaking:

1. A bedroom is the place where we sleep. It is also the place where much of the discussion about uncomfortable topics takes place. Many married couples with children choose to avoid confrontation during the day, in order to safeguard the feelings of their children. At night though, the bedroom becomes the battlefield for discussion, and in some cases, fights. The result in this case is that the couple spends nights lying back to back to each other, with feelings of anger and hurt. Not good for love.

2. The bed is the number-one place for discussing. . .MONEY.

3. The bedroom is one of those neutral spaces, where little is done

to make the interior personalized, beautiful, and happy. It is one of those rooms that gets furnished once in a lifetime and that's it. We are much more likely to replace the couch in our living room than buy a new bed or soft bed linen, or rearrange the location of the (sinking) love vessel.

4. Lighting is another neglected item in many bedrooms. Reading lights, those nasty little light bulbs placed right and left of our beds, are a disaster. We have the power to control them independently, which sends a clear signal to the person next to us. Light on, leave me alone I want to read. Light off, leave me alone I want to sleep. "Leave me alone" is the message.

5. When was the last time you changed the pictures or art on the walls of your bedroom? Well? Photographs from holidays taken a million years ago, in a bikini, dress the walls of the room in which we change from our work clothes into our PJ's every night. No tan, no palm trees to enhance our silhouettes. There are also pictures of children and family members. It doesn't get any less exciting than this.

Are you convinced yet about the destructive powers of our bedrooms, if we leave them unattended for too long? Attention is what they need. A little TLC and a shared plan to make this room into a true nest will do the trick. So step No. 1 to transform the bedroom from a sinking old vessel into a fine cruise ship is this:

Think Beautiful Thoughts, and Invest in Them

This is an important part of the Sex-Rehabilitation-for-Body-Workers Rescue Plan. We need to invest (thus spending some money), in the new venture. In a way, we have to gear ourselves up for this.

First stop is a hardware store. Yes, a hardware store. You can get dimmers in a variety of price ranges, and they will make a huge difference in your new bedroom. Experiment with different light bulbs too. Blue, red, or yellow are nice light-diffusing colors that give skin a beautiful texture and invite touch.

Lighting also brings up a point that must be as old as the invention of electricity. Men like to make love with the lights on. Women hate it. I bet you there was much more love making going on when candles were around and bright overhead lights weren't an option.

For the best sexy lighting, we should place the light on the floor, in a corner, or under the bed. In filmmaking, it's called "indirect, diffused light." And guess what: it is used for love scenes. Best of all, your partner is the one who needs to install the dimmer. It is his or her contribution to gearing up for your new love life. It is certainly much nicer to install a dimmer when your thoughts revolve around body pleasures, than installing a dimmer in the kitchen or your kid's bedroom.

Next in order of importance is buying new bed linen. There are beautiful microfiber fabrics out there, in a variety of colors. Pick one that you like. Have your partner pick the other one.

This is all about NOT compromising. This is about reclaiming individual identity, which is why people fall in love in the first place. It is because we find interest in each other that we would like to explore. We are trying to create a place that feels foreign, inviting, and stimulating.

Take any crazy Vegas hotel, with revolving heart-shaped beds in bright pink or red. They don't furnish their interiors with grandma's inherited bedding, washed a million times, with a few buttons missing here and there. Why? Because it screams carelessness, boredom, and tiredness from miles away. Replace the linen, create a new environment, and use this symbol of love and attention as an anchor to announce your intention for change.

The environment plays a huge part in our ability to relax, let go, and accept.

Buy some candles and essential oils. You can add a little scent to your pillows. Ylang-ylang, for instance, is known for aphrodisiac powers, but you could also use any fragrance that feels good to you, aphrodisiac or not. Buy a new CD, and if you have no sound-producing device in your bedroom, get an inexpensive CD player. Music is amazing, music is personal, music is a backdrop to your personality and gives atmosphere (and—ahem—rhythm) to your love life.

Transforming the Nest

Now you are ready to go home and make it happen. Take your time. Sit down. Get some wine or coffee and just sit. Look at your bedroom, and say goodbye. Take a deep breath and throw every single piece of dirty clothing, along with the laundry basket and everything that feels boring, out of that room. Now explore different bed positioning options. If you have windows and it is warm enough, place the bed under the window and organize the pillows so that you are actually able to look outside. Can you see the sky? At night, gazing at the moon and the stars is a good setting for an intimate, caring talk.

Change the bed linen, find a good place for your new lights, and distribute the candles. Write a little card to your loved one. Explain what this means to you. Let him or her discover the makeover by him or herself. You will know how to work the details of your bedroom and relationship renaissance.

Then email me and tell me how it went!

Family Matters

Family members, and often friends too, have the tendency to regard our work as a hobby. One of hardest things to do is to explain, without sounding too diva-ish, that we can not "quickly" show them a few exercises, teaching a private session between chairs, tables, running televisions, screaming infants, and the occasional cell phone call, without compromising what the Pilates craft is all about: concentration, awareness, and attention to form and detail.

That's right! Our work is not a hobby, it is a profession. On top of the requirements that any profession includes, such as time, finance, facility management, reaching sales targets, (and the list goes on), our job deals with people—people who come to us for wellness require a specific set of human qualities: empathy, willingness to listen, ability to share. Providing these qualities, if not monitored, depletes our energy reservoir.

Energizing is People-Specific

Energy is the most valuable asset we have. It is not endless; it needs to be fuelled. We all fuel ourselves in different ways.

"When I get home, I do not want to talk to anybody for at least thirty minutes," says Elizabeth Larkam. "Even when I have a cancellation and a colleague comes along for a chat, I wish I could put up a sign that reads: Not open to the public."

Some of us recharge through isolation, and others recharge through human contact. A male Pilates teacher reported that the thirty-minute drive from the studio to home was his time out, where he could be silent and get some distance from his teaching day. Sometimes working far away from home creates a space that allows us to detach from the role of teacher into the one of partner and family member. Still, we need to learn how our partners operate. It is important to know how our partners recharge and to respect their space.

We can all see the potential problem here. Pilates teacher who needs isolation to recharge (intrinsic energizing) comes home from his or her studio and is greeted by a partner who can't wait to pour out all his thoughts and happenings in order to recharge his own batteries (extrinsic energizing). Result? The intrinsic energizer is less than excited about the information overload that she is a experiencing and gets grumpy, which in turn annoys the extrinsic energizer.

At least our family members or partners are close by. We see them at night and talk to them regularly. What about the other facet of human interaction, friendships?

Friendship = Less Stress = Better Health

This profession can make us isolated even though we bathe daily in a sea of people, in sounds, smells, and information; at night, the last thing I am able to do is call a far-away friend on the phone for an extended chat or talk to my partner about my day. TV is often the answer. In order to replenish and receive after a long day of primary giving to others, I end up sitting in front of a television.

"In terms of friendship for my part, there are not really any real, close friends that I am able to give time to," says Brent Anderson, CEO of Polestar Pilates. "So many great people extend their friendship to me, but I usually have to decline. When I am home I want to spend time with my family. It's a choice you make."

What about men in the mind-body profession? I have not forgotten you! But I believe that Pilates men are a species of their own. Are they more in touch with themselves and others, more sensitive maybe?

Some men I spoke to were in line with the common assumption that men see friendship differently than women do. Men are less likely to turn to friends immediately when they are stressed. As a result, men appear to be more likely than women to suffer stress's harmful effects, which may be due to their lack of willingness to share their problems. They do not befriend others as much as women do. They have no outlet and get tired and stressed, often becoming sick as a result.

These are gender-related coping strategies. Women are more likely to turn to friends; men are more likely to exhibit "fight or flight."

Tend and Befriend

Research at UCLA on friendship and stress reports that women automatically turn to friends in response to stressful situations. This pattern is called "tend and befriend" due to the natural response of women to tend to their young, thus protecting them, and befriend by seeking support from others.

The other coping behavior is called "fight or flight." Both genders can exhibit the "fight or flight" responses. We confront the problem or disappear to escape from it, thereby missing out on the beneficial activity of dividing the burden of the problem with people who like us.

The sum of all these considerations is basically this: We do not have unlimited amounts of energy; nobody does. If we run ourselves down too much, replenishing becomes difficult and our fine, oriental mind-body rug will start to wear thin.

Relationships are the most important things we have in our lives. We are nothing without them. We also have responsibilities toward those around us. One of these is taking care of ourselves so we can be there for them.

We have to practice what we preach. If this means making less money because we are teaching fewer classes, than so be it. After all, we will have a lifetime of energy to slowly pay back our monetary debt. But it's easier and nicer to do this when we are happy.

Now, go buy that light.

8

Healthy Teaching

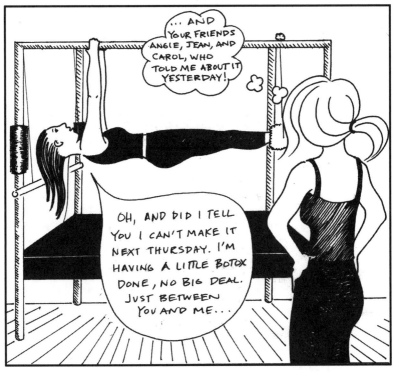

Confidentiality Clause

Myth Versus Reality? How Fit We Really Are

Our clients really, honestly believe that we work out every day, for several hours, on all pieces of equipment. We wish!

The reality of a busy studio schedule is that it leaves little time for workouts: most trainers report seeing between six and eight clients per day plus the additional mat classes. We are lucky if we make it onto the equipment three times per week.

The lack of regular training combined with the need to demonstrate exercises without proper warm up can be injury inducing and is not good for our bodies. Like school teachers, Pilates trainers live in a breeding ground for all sorts of illnesses, from influenza to chicken pox to herpes. If we would cancel a session every time we feel sick, we could not survive—it is hard enough to make up for client cancellations at the last minute. Taking care of ourselves to prevent illness and to get through it if it happens is paramount.

As in many other jobs, teaching Pilates involves a fair amount of repetitive movement. We bend over a lot, handle equipment, assist in stretches, change springs, are exposed to illness, and talk constantly. These are only a few of the physical stressors that affect Pilates teachers.

Psychologically, we also gear ourselves up to listen to and support clients in life mishaps and joys; sometimes we teach clients who we do not really like, we have to keep anger in check if clients do not pay or cancel constantly, and we deal with loss when clients who we are very fond of move or become seriously ill. There are issues that relate to the organization or studio for which we work. We interact with co-workers, we probably work under a boss, and sometimes our teaching philosophies do not entirely blend with the organizational culture of the studio.

These areas have been studied in a line of research called "ergonomics." The word is Greek: "ergo" means work; "nomos" means laws.

Ergonomic Teaching

We have all heard of ergonomics and probably picture herds of physical therapists strolling through offices trying to teach workers how to more healthily spend eight hours per day on the computer by adjusting their screens, tables, and chairs. But ergonomics are much more than that. The Human Factors and Ergonomics Society of Australia has a good description of what this field entails. Ergonomics essentially refer to human factors, anything that affects us, physically, psychologically, and socially, during our jobs.

I. Physical Ergonomics

Physical ergonomics deals with the human anatomical, physiological, and biomechanical characteristics of our work. The most commonly mentioned physical stressors of the Pilates teachers I interviewed were the following:

Lack of Natural Light

We have to realize that spending time inside all day, often with no natural light, is energy draining in itself. In fact, spending so much time inside presents considerable health hazards.

The National Institute of Health Clinical Center Web site tells us vitamin D is responsible for maintaining healthy levels of calcium and phosphorus in our blood. Helping calcium to be absorbed, Vitamin D makes our bones strong. Sources of vitamin D include certain foods and exposure to sunlight. It is suggested that there appears to be a correlation between lack of vitamin D and osteoporosis.

Populations that are especially at risk for vitamin D deficiency include people living in the northern hemisphere where there are just not enough hours of sunlight for our bodies to be exposed to (such as Alaska or Scandinavia), menopausal women, and generally speaking, anybody over the age of 50 who spends a lot of time inside. Regardless, whether we are teachers in our 20's or 40's, long-term, our job makes us susceptible to Vitamin D deficiency-related problems. In order to avoid vitamin D deficiency and to break up our days, we should try to combine time spent outside with a good diet.

Do we need to bake in sun for hours? Of course not, but it is suggested to spend at least a few minutes outside every day. Lack of sunshine has very direct effects on our psyche as well.

"Try to get out and take a walk when you have a break," Eva Powers, a Stott Pilates instructor teacher tells her trainees "The lack of fresh air and sunlight can be very energy consuming."

In terms of diet, we should make sure to include fish (salmon, mackerel, sardines), milk (nonfat, reduced fat, whole, or vitamin D fortified), cereal grain bars, dry cereal, and eggs, just to name a few key foods. The best way to look at this is to make sure that we eat well and regularly and make time for an outside walk during the day. Choosing exercise outside of Pilates that takes place outdoors is also very helpful. Cycling, rollerblading, and running are all good ways to get out and integrate cardiovascular training as well as some fresh air into our lives.

These activities can be problematic if we suffer from injuries. Some of them can directly result from our non-ergonomic teaching practices.

1. Changing Springs and Bending Over

There were several injuries mentioned that appeared to be directly related to the repetitive action of changing springs. Effected areas included hands, wrists, and shoulder girdles. Several teachers reported being diagnosed with carpal tunnel syndrome.

The spring problem can be easily remedied. Changing springs is only problematic if we do so bending around the corner of a machine. If we stand in front of the foot bar and manipulate the springs with the body in alignment, wrist, hand, and shoulder problems should be in check. Moira Merrithew suggests the following: "The easiest way to avoid changing springs as often is to teach clients to do it themselves," she says. "Of course this only works if they have been working with you for a while and are not injured."

I tried it myself and found that clients actually quite enjoy doing it, because they get a good feeling for the spring load and how it relates to different muscle groups. Another action that can cause lower back pain is the constant bending over in order to align, correct, or assist in stretches. Even if we try to have good alignment, our focus is directed downward. Since most of us have good posture in terms of our thoracic spine alignment, we are very likely to hinge from our lower backs. Our own body proportions need to be taken into consideration as well, in order to make teaching ergonomic.

For example, if I am five feet, one inch in height with long legs and a short torso, the leverage on my lower back is less than that experienced by a six foot tall teacher with a long torso and short legs. If we were able to adjust the Reformer or Trapeze Table in height once the client is on these machines, this would greatly improve the physical ergonomics of our workplace because our posture would be more dynamic.

I was really grateful to Pilates equipment manufactures when they put wheels on the Reformer because it made the equipment so much nicer to maneuver. Kristopher Bosch and Dan Burke, who are physical therapists and own a studio in Buffalo, New York, also laughed about the weight of the new ladder barrel they just acquired. "It is so heavy that lugging it around becomes a workout in itself! It's great for the client—the apparatus is more stable," Dan says, "but not for US!"

How about a nice hydraulic pump to adjust the height of the Trapeze or the Reformer? A set of retractable wheels for the ladder barrel and the chair?

Elizabeth Larkam chose a different route. "I used to kneel all the time because the reformer and trapeze table are so low," says Elizabeth

Larkam,: "Let me tell you, I had holes in the knees of some of my pants!"

It seems to me that any other professional who is required to bend over for his or her job, such as chiropractors, dentists, or massage therapists, has a choice of several body-friendly tools in order to protect their own health as well as their clients'.

Dear manufacturers! Maybe now you would possibly consider helping us out and creating some fabulous new design—we can't wait! Meanwhile, can we make teaching more body friendly for ourselves? Yes, we can.

Elizabeth has more good advice. "We should make sure to wear comfortable shoes and use physio balls to sit on. When I taught at St. Francis Hospital, we used rolling stools from the medical school. Boy were they great to scoot around on!"

So making sure that we move around even when seated is paramount in order to create a dynamic postural pattern. It is also very good for the client: if we just check them from one angle we cannot always tell what is going on. Walking around constantly is one of the things I really took to heart from my own training with Eva Powers. In the exam, you actually got points taken off if you did not do it enough!

2. Injuries Due to Poor Warm-Up

Since we are teaching exercises and good teaching requires a certain amount of modeling, at some point during the class, we are likely to get down on the mat or equipment and show an exercise. This is when a lot of injuries happen, especially when you have a client who is working above the beginning level on the equipment or on the mat. Warming up before we start to teach is very important for our bodies. We check in with ourselves and make a mental note of problematic areas. We become aware. We need a warm-up just like anybody else does.

Eva Powers believes that just a couple of exercises in order to ground ourselves and get ready for the task ahead are very beneficial.

Getting to the session in a hurry with the client waiting is not very good. Arriving 15 minutes early for our first clients of the day is not only professional, but gives us a chance to do at least one brief exercise before we get going and focus on our clients. Our preparation is important for both us and them.

Warming up with our clients on the mat is another good strategy to take in order to tune in with our bodies and get ready for possibly more challenging demonstrations later on. It is with our intermediate and advances clients that this is going to be particularly crucial—demonstrating a full swan dive requires preparation. In any case, we should always do a few preps. Use the preps as a tool to reinforce the different stages of mastering an exercise. I will never forget how my first instructor teacher Trent McEntire always did three to five preparations before he would show us the full swan dive. He modeled care on his own body and it stuck with me.

Lynne Robinson chooses another good way to reduce the risk of injury. "I try to do some of the warm-up alongside the client and tailor my own workout a little differently after a long teaching day." She says "Since we are more likely to demonstrate abdominal exercises in flexion than in extension, my own workout really focuses on this area." Again, balancing is key.

3. Voice

We have seen that there are things we can do to improve our teaching routine. Voice, however, is a whole other kettle of fish. Voice problems are CAREER THREATENING. I kid you not! For instance, in our beginnings as teachers, when we are likely to teach endless amounts of mat classes, our voices will give in if we do not take care of them. The population primarily at risk here is actually the very experienced teachers, those who lead workshops and certification courses. Their voice never gets a rest because they are likely to teach through a week-end and dive right into their weekly schedule without a break.

Lindsay Merrithew is an actor by "trade": "I can absolutely see the value of voice training for Pilates teachers," he says. "Actors have voice training to make it through a run and this area is considered essential for their profession."

The issue of voice training is therefore especially meaningful to consider if you are an instructor trainer. The amount of constant talking over several days can be harmful and needs to be trained to sustain such teaching marathons. These hazards can be reduced through simple measures, if we are made aware of them. I would argue that raising awareness of the importance of good voice placement should be part of every teacher training, and regular coaching could be offered on the subject at conferences on a regular basis.

Kornelia Ritterpusch, who studied Pilates with Alan Herdman in London, was one of the first to open a Pilates studio in Germany, fifteen years ago. Kornelia started having problems with her voice when she was about five years into her professional teaching career. Weekend Pilates seminars, where she was expected to talk constantly for two days, started her path to serious vocal cord problems and pulmonary infections that have been with her until today.

Kornelia told me that there is a true downward spiral to a future of voice problems.

It usually all begins with the "common" sore throat. We feel a slight tingling in our throat and think nothing of it. Since we have committed to our teaching load, we ignore these symptoms and. . .keep talking.

The vocal cords, already irritated and inflamed, are easy targets for infections, which lead to a partial or full loss of voice. Now we take medication while we teach, but again, professionals that we are, we keep talking.

Then things get worse, because we do actually get severely sick. Chronic laryngitis, pulmonary infections, and other respiratory tract illnesses become frequent companions. We now need to cancel some classes. We feel guilty, and sooner than recommended, we resume teaching and. . .keep talking.

The downward spiral never stops. Once throat infections become chronic, we are likely to take antibiotics regularly. These help us get back on track, but have weakening repercussions on the immune system, which in turn triggers other infections. "I have had lots of trouble with my voice, and the thing to remember is to keep your throat wet, small sips of water," says Lynne Robinson. "If you have music going, turn it down. Teach small classes. The Body Control Pilates Code of Practice limits classes to twelve clients max. Bring your clients in closer to you."

The message is this: a simple sore throat can become an existence-threatening problem that takes many days out of our teaching schedules. Voice problems are so blatantly obvious that everybody will know that we are sick. After a while, they will start wondering what this all about. Before we know it, we are building ourselves a reputation for being sickly and weak. We have to address the problem with professional help.

The reasons that we may use our voices the wrong ways can have several roots. One is self esteem, and another is training.

Our voice gives a lot of information on our emotional state and how comfortable we feel leading a class in front of people. Public speaking can be one of the most anxiety-inducing activities. In fact, if researchers need to get people's heart rates up, the easiest way to do it is to tell them that they have to speak in front of people and that they have five minutes to prepare. Wham! Heart rate goes up, pupils react, the whole nine yards of physical reactions to arousal happens in a heartbeat.

Teaching is public speaking. Any teaching engagement is more or less challenging depending on our comfort level. Our voices react to the stress. No matter how experienced we are, our voices reflect what we think and feel.

Again, we need to warm up. Hum on your way to work—put on a nice song and sing along to it; sing in the shower—the humidity of the water cascading down warms up your throat and loosens any residue.

Inhalation with essential oils is also wonderful. It clears the head and disinfects the breathing passages. All we need is hot (not boiling!) water, a few drops of eucalyptus or tea tree oil, and a towel. Put two oil drops in a large bowl and pour the water over it. Then wait a few seconds for it to cool down and place your head over the bowl and a towel over your head. Breathe deeply; try to stay for about ten minutes. Enjoy!

The second reason for voice problems is that we do not get coaching for voice. Taking singing lessons or working with a vocal coach gives us access to the workings of the diaphragm and how we can use our voices in an energy-saving manner. If we only use our throat voices, our diaphragms do not move. We are essentially making sounds without support, much like doing exercises without core control. Kornelia Ritterpusch, who has been working with a vocal coach for years, suggests the following to safeguard our voices:

- We have to hear ourselves speak. We must make an active effort to evaluate the tone and pitch of our voices and be attuned to them.

- We should speak with a chest voice instead of a throat voice. How do we know which one we are generally using? Here is a good exercise, taken from the British Vocalist Organization:

Place two fingers on your breast bone and start humming a tone starting from the deepest note you can possibly produce. Then sing your way up the scale. When you feel vibrations in your hand, you know you are using your chest voice. As you go up the scale into the higher notes, for which you will use your head voice, the vibration will take place somewhere between your lips and your forehead.

Now say something normally, in your usual speaking voice, still keeping the fingers on your breastbone. Does it vibrate? No? Welcome to the club of people who speak in their head voices, thus straining their vocal cords! Practice teaching in your chest voice every day from now on. It will feel so much easier than speaking in your head voice. Your voice will be less high-pitched (which, by the way, is distracting and comes across as strained or frantic), and will have a warm, comforting sound to it.

- Our voices also need to be supported by breath. Breathe slowly as you teach, and pace yourself. This is a completely different way of breathing than what we teach in a Pilates class, but it sends oxygen into our backs and stomachs and allows the diaphragm to support us as we speak. Not breathing the Pilates way, i.e., breathing into our stomachs instead of our sides, is very good for us when we speak. Trainers hold a lot more tension in their core than the recommended 20% to 30% which is needed to balance our skeletal system. Partly, we do this for cosmetic reasons, since clients expect us to have a solid core, and breathing into our stomachs will let this area relax and stick out. I also feel that we often do the exercises with our clients and tense up our own body parts to "help them" through an exercise. When I started teaching, I stored a lot of tension in my rotators and glutei muscles and wondered why at night my sacrum felt so tight. Now I try to breathe into my stomach actively, and I often stand in medial rotation to relax the lower back and legs. Not very attractive, but it helps a lot!

4. Health Risks

Working in a studio means constant interaction with and exposure to bacteria and viruses. This is why it is so important to clean mats and equipment after they have been used.

Viruses, bacteria, and other pathogens enter our body in numerous ways: through our respiratory or digestive systems, or breaks in our skin, for example. Washing our hands between every class is very helpful in reducing the spread of colds and influenza. We should also consider encouraging clients to cancel if they think that they are getting a cold or have children at home with infectious diseases.

Lynne goes even further: "I am adamant about canceling sessions if I am sick or if they are sick. And no sick children in the corner. And take time out for yourself. We give all day—do something where you are given to, like a massage or a facial or a class for yourself."

We need to be especially careful if we have a large number of pregnant women taking class in the studio. Putting up a sign asking for collaboration at the beginning of the fall and throughout the winter can help keep us healthier. Even here, essential oils can be useful in disinfecting the room at the beginning of a teaching day, and it is good to open the windows (if you have them) for fresh air after classes.

5. Teaching Out

Ergonomic teaching practices are especially important if we make house calls. House calls are often warranted with older people who may be scared to leave their houses in the winter or simply do not want to make their way to the studio. The problem is that teaching a mat class to people who do not have much control over their weight and movement is downright dangerous for the teacher. If someone falls onto me with full body weight in order to get down on the mat, I need all my strength to be of assistance.

Let me give you one example. My studio partner was approached by a condominium group to offer Pilates classes as part of their renter-friendly services. The class is free for the clients, but we get paid by the session.

First of all, these people had no idea what Pilates was because they had not been informed. They arrived with sneakers and towels only to find that they were expected to lie down on an ice cold, marble floor. My partner was further expected to move half a dozen tables out of the way, and move these back to their original locations when she was done. On top of all that, the people in this mat class had serious physical issues. One person had recently had a double hip replacement, another one had cerebral palsy, the next one had knee pain.

Those of us who work in a studio exclusively are really lucky! But there are hundreds of teachers who do home calls or teach in churches or other facilities that can be downright atrocious to work in. We need to be assertive about our working conditions. It is our bodies on the line, and as we all know, those we cannot exchange.

Eight hours of teaching per day for months on end will do anybody's back in, hydraulic pump or not. Doing the same exercises without change gets boring and loses its purpose if we are not motivated. Injuries that we thought were long resolved will flare up if we allow ourselves to be idle and play the "I am a Pilates teacher but I don't need to do Pilates anymore" game.

The easiest way to protect ourselves and teach effectively is to work out DAILY. Many of us are or have been injured; that's how we came to Pilates in the first place. We need to attend to our injuries, and this means doing the work. Every time I slack off in terms of training, my back acts up immediately. My body feels out of tune and I don't feel good.

So, I wondered, what do the Pilates superstars think about this?

Elizabeth Larkam works out all the time, and you can tell that she does. "Our bodies need to be finely tuned instruments in order to teach effectively" says Elizabeth "and the only way to keep going is to practice and invest the money that we make in our own bodywork community. I have several standing appointments with practitioners per week."

Rael Isacowitz is another master teacher who believes in doing the work, always.

"Practice is crucial," Rael says. "I spend so much time on planes and at airports, leading workshops from China to South Africa, Europe, Australia, and the United States. But I practice daily: it is part of my being, like eating or breathing. Not practicing cannot be justified, for any reason; being busy is not a reason, travel is not a reason. One must practice to be true and credible, and to work with integrity."

After surviving the physical ergonomics section, we now proceed to the psychological aspects of being a Pilates teacher.

II. Cognitive Ergonomics

These ergonomics are related to mental aptitudes such as perception, decision making, and mental workload. They relate to mental stuff, which often times is completely irrational and very hard to change.

1. Perception

Are our perceptions of our clients accurate? Are we always attentive to the things we say and what kind of reactions they may provoke? Dealing with bodies is tricky, because people tend to be very vulnerable about criticism or suggestions for improvement related to their physiques or, even worse, their mental states. Depending on the personality who is in front of you, a well-meant comment can trigger responses that are totally disproportionate.

In her book *The Educated Heart: Professional Guidelines for Massage Therapists, Bodyworkers and Movement Teachers*, Nina McIntosh discusses the imbalance of power that is inherent in the Therapist/Client relationship. Due to the nature of the relationship, we the trainers are placed in a position of power that we have to be careful not to exploit. Believe it or not, our clients really listen to us! They take comments, tweak them in their heads to fit their particular mind sets (we all do this!) and run with it. The most dangerous facet of this is when we abuse our role as teachers and claim to have expertise in other areas.

We have all heard trainers placing themselves in the role of the therapist. Phrases such as, "My client is really opening up, she cried during the session," or, "My client told me about her terrible divorce and felt much better after our session," come from well-intentioned teachers but are absolutely out of line. If we are not trained as psychologists or social workers, and do not have any other counseling training, we should refrain from giving psychological advice. Period.

For one, we cannot make a reliable diagnosis regarding mental conditions, let alone treat them. Furthermore, we put ourselves in a vulnerable position when we have to come to terms with the information itself. Last but not least, private information pertaining to family members who you may be training as well puts you in the hot seat. One wrong action and you are toast, no matter how well-intentioned the action was initially.

2. Decision Making

If you find yourself bending the rules for a particular client all the time, such as consistently not charging late cancellation fees, allowing unreasonable schedule changes, extending the session well beyond the hour, or making financial allowances even though you can't afford it, those are red flags. Think about it right now. Isn't it always the same clients who give you a headache? Who cancel three times out of five? Who pay late or not at all? Who forget their appointments? Who seem to think that all you do, all day long is wait for them to make up their minds on when they would like to work out? Conversations with them go like this: "Maybe tomorrow at 6, or Thursday at 8AM; actually, that week I am on vacation, so it would be great if we could do Sunday night at 10."

Or how about this scenario: It is Sunday night, you had a fantastic weekend, and you look at your Monday schedule. Ugh. There it is: the dreaded name. Within a second, you feel five tons of weight on your shoulders.

These are essentially decision-making situations. Ask yourself, do I really need this client? Would I not rather invest my energy into someone who is eager to learn and less demanding? The energy these people take out of you ("Energy Suckers," as Brent Anderson calls them) is not worth it.

Look out for red flags when you meet new clients.

The easiest way to identify red flags according to studio owner Nancy Hodari is to listen to your client. Nancy claims that "even if you are just starting up and in need of business, it is important to make sure that we evaluate the starting pointers of a new client relationship. Do they criticize everyone they have ever worked with? Well, you are probably in for trouble and better let that chunk of business go. It will cost you a lot of anguish and stress to work with someone that negative, and the chances are that he or she will bad mouth you just the same way in a few weeks' time."

We can probably deal with one or two clients who qualify as energy suckers if we keep them well within their boundaries and have many other wonderful clients to look forward to. If the "suckers" take over, we need to take action immediately. Reduce their hours. Only seeing them once a week will do wonders for our psyches!

3. Workload

How much teaching can we do, and do well?

"Generally speaking, teaching four clients back to back calls for a break." Says Eva Powers "This is important for both parties because the trainer is tired after four hours of intense concentration and can not possibly give the client the attention he deserves long after this. Obviously though, this is a personal matter."

Within limits, teaching at different places and seeing different people is good and gets us out of a routine. Keeping diversity in our scheduling if possible, in order to make each day a little different, is also energizing. A very heavy day could be followed by a lighter one, and two days off a week help us replenish. We need time to read a book, take other classes, and "vacuum out" the mind; this should be top priority if your schedule looks like a tornado of classes, workshops, and business meetings!

Burnout: Are You at Risk?

Clients can tell if we are tired. Monotonous voice, lack of creativity in the programming of exercises, and barely having the strength, zest, or interest to walk around someone, let alone assisting him or her in a stretch, are all prime indicators of overload. The best possible check to see if you may be suffering from this is the following question. How often do you check your watch during class time? I know someone who checks hers in three minute intervals—I am so aware of it now that when I teach, I avoid looking at my watch if the client can see me. Sometimes checking the time in order to program effectively is called for. But if you are really in the moment and interested in what you are doing, this should not happen constantly. Does the clock rule your life? Can you not wait to get out of the studio?

Many teachers experience this. Troy McCarty, an internationally renowned ballet master and owner of three successful studios in Ohio brought this up when I was telling him about the book. "Are you going to talk about burnout? Because three years ago, running three studios, spending hours in car and on the phone, I had just about had it!"

Burnout syndrome is a stress condition. If we work too much, put pressure on ourselves or take pressure from others for too long, our bodies shut down. We have no energy, lack interest in what we used to passionate about, and can't take anymore. When I researched suggestions for avoiding or fighting burnout, the overall suggestion from academics is almost laughable: Lie down and breathe, relax, take a mind-body fitness class (now there is a joke!), and redefine your role in life.

Redefining our roles in life? How does that work?

John Sealey, a communication coach based in Hamburg, Germany, went through all of it himself when he quit a high-paying job to do his own thing: "Work means different things to different people. When was the last time you stood back from work, far enough away, in fact, to ask yourself what your job actually means to you? How well does it fit with the other things that make up the wonderful jigsaw puzzle of your life?" Ask yourself:

- Do you see your work as a means to an end? Paying the bills, the mortgage?

- Have you turned your favorite pastime into your profession? And if you did is it still what you hoped it to be?

- Would you rather be doing something else instead?

- Is it the challenge that gives you that special buzz every time you get up in the morning?

"There are no wrong or right answers here," John says. "We all have different motivators for the work we do. But perhaps the interesting question to ask yourself is if what you do fits in with who you are and the way you wish to lead your life. Is it authentic for you?"

Troy told me that his moment of burnout was probably due a combination of events: too much work, a less-than-ideal partnership, and the wish to explore other talents. "Teaching ballet really helps me balance my work in the Pilates studio." He says "I could not teach only Pilates anymore."

Since most of us came to Pilates through different routes, we could perhaps consider integrating an aspect of our previous jobs that we really enjoyed. It all comes back to balance.

III. Organizational Ergonomics

The third element of ergonomics is ergonomics of the organization for which we work. Essentially, this relates to whether we feel valued and rewarded in our profession, whether we know what is expected of us, and whether we trained specifically in those areas that require further development. Since it deals with larger groups of people, this section is geared toward studio owners or Pilates corporations.

These considerations are relevant for teachers who work for big Pilates organizations or in large studios, but also for the soloists in how they keep up communication with their certifying organizations.

Dr. Gerrit Knodt, a Human Resource professor at the Ecole de Management in Nantes, France, truly believes the old saying that "people are our greatest assets." A quick glance at the literature on transfer of learning shows us that that the transfer from trainees knowing things (which can be tested in an exam) to them actually applying this knowledge on the job is disturbingly low.

On top of that, it is also clear that a huge amount of learning occurs on the job. The quality of this behavior, however, often reinforces past behaviors and attitudes rather then promoting new ones. Essentially, what we learn on the job is to do things just how everybody else in our immediate environment does things. We perpetuate the status quo, following the maxim: "We have always done it this way!" We are wrong if we think that knowing something (cognitive state) and doing something (behavioral state) is the same thing.

Dr. Knodt says that the fundamental principles underlying training and development are not hard to identify. If you have employees and wonder why they are not motivated or seem to have problems implementing what you expect of them, you may want to look at this checklist closely.

Did you. . .

- Select the right people for the right jobs?

- Teach people the things they need to know to do their jobs?

- Reinforce teaching with assessment and feedback?

- Objectively measure performance?

- Reward performance when it is good?

- Put into place consequences when performance is consistently poor?

Bottom line and tool extraordinaire is this: what gets taught, measured, and rewarded has excellent chances of being done and enjoyed.

Training and development is part of our health and happiness. In his book, *Return to Life through Contrology* Joseph Pilates, said:

"Physical fitness is the first requisite of happiness. Our interpretation of physical fitness is the attainment and maintenance of a uniformly developed body with a sound mind fully capable of naturally, easily, and satisfactorily performing our many and varied daily tasks with spontaneous zest and pleasure."

We mustn't forget to have fun!

9

Mentorship: The "Dying Bug" Is Going to Hamburg

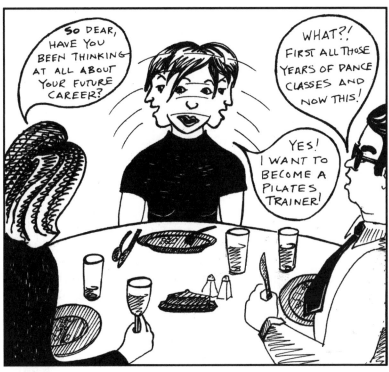

Pilates Career

Last year, I moved to another country and began looking for a teacher a few days after I had settled into my house. I had heard about my potential mentor, Khita Whyatt, for quite some time, because she has been a Pilates and Rolfing practitioner since 1986, when most people didn't even know how "Pilates" was spelled, let alone what it was.

Khita was extremely gracious from the beginning, and I could only gasp at her immense knowledge of functional anatomy, which she was nonchalantly mentioning in conjunction with exercises. Khita trains Pilates instructors and has developed many variations of traditional exercises herself, naming them depending on their qualities or looks. One variation for the abdominal muscles that she taught me is called the "dying bug."

One day, I dragged a visiting German friend of mine to her studio to take class. I had taught her some of Khita's exercises during my last visit—the "dying bug," of course, among others. So I said: "By the way, I have taught my friend some of your exercises, so now the dying bug is going to Hamburg." Khita replied: "As long as I am going with him, that's great!"

Khita and I had discussed at length the issues of intellectual property regarding exercises. How do you protect your ideas in relationship to movement?

Khita, a Native American, pointed out to me that the Western notion of "copyright" is really alien to her. In her own culture, sharing information with others is one of the ways it gets protected, being passed down from generation to generation through mentorship. As a mentee you take pride in showing respect to those who taught you by acknowledging them.

We have to acknowledge the sources when we use other people's information in our classes. In the mind-body community, so many details are passed on from Joseph Pilates' students themselves (also called first-generation teachers) that this heritage should be part of our philosophy and integrate in our teachings.

Lineage gives historical support to what we do and helps establish each of our Pilates self-conceptions. Adding the sources of what moves and influences us in our classes is our responsibility if we want the same courtesy extended to us by our own students.

Certain elements of good teaching are universal, and one of these all-important elements is having mentors that advise, guide, and inspire us.

Mentorship

In the early Greek world, all education functioned in terms of mentorship. You found someone who could not only teach you the secrets and details of your craft, but who could assume a leadership role and help you grow into your profession. Today, most Pilates education is organized in weekend workshops, where you may find an instructor who is right in line with your Pilates philosophy, or you may not. When you return to your home studio, you are on your own, most likely relying on your colleagues to gather new information about exercises, modifications, equipment, and the like.

Mentors are few and far between. They are individuals who have many years of experience in their professions and are willing to share their expertise with others. They are generous yet firm, charismatic and creative. They never stop learning, and this is what makes them unique: since they are on a permanent mission to learn anyway, they will welcome any opportunity to share their knowledge with us, because five seconds later they are on to the next thing. I also believe that with many years of experience, mentors start "connecting the dots"; things make sense on a bigger, visionary level.

Everybody I spoke to had at least one mentor. For Rael Isacowitz, there have been many teachers from the methods of dance and yoga who have influenced him deeply. He studied with all of the first-generation teachers at some point in his life, but he feels a special, charismatic relationship with Kathy Grant. Here is his account:

Getting "Undressed on the Wunder Chair"

Rael Isacowitz, Founder and Director of Body Arts and Science International

Unfortunately, I have not had one specific mentor who I studied with for a long period of time. I had wonderful teachers in dance, yoga, and my many athletic pursuits.

I have studied Pilates, or at the very least taken sessions with most of the Pilates "elders." I would say though, that I have a very special rapport, trust, and chemistry with Kathy Grant.

I will never forget when I first started working with her on the Wunder Chair. At this point, I already had years of experience doing Pilates, I was an accomplished professional dancer, I had a masters degree in dance and human movement, and felt like I had mastered the most complex repertoire in the Pilates method.

Kathy then asked me to demonstrate an exercise on the Wunder Chair. (Joseph Pilates had worked extensively with Kathy on the Wunder Chair, which gave her invaluable and innate knowledge of this apparatus and the body in general.)

Well, metaphorically speaking, she completely "undressed" me. Her insightful critique made me completely reevaluate my work!

I had to let go of my protection, my ego, my bravado—whatever you want to call it. It was hard initially, but ultimately I reaped the rewards. It taught me to truly work from the inside out. Although I was performing the most advanced repertoire, I was really thinking of choreography, not controlled movement emanating from deep within.

She had such a profound influence on me and really set my teaching and practicing on a new path, a path that has taught me the infinite possibilities of this work.

□ □ □

Being a good mentor to many students over the years sometimes turns a person into a "master teacher." Since masters seem to be popping up at every local studio, I figured that it may be important to clarify what being a master entails and how we can discern a real master teacher from those who may be a little further away from this high goal. Again, for this section I turned to Rael, undisputedly a Pilates master.

Niki: "Rael, everybody wants to be a master teacher these days. How is a master teacher different from a regular instructor trainer? Is a master teacher more about conveying the philosophy of Pilates or about teaching the method?"

Rael: "I think that it is BOTH and much, much more than that. The term 'master' teacher has been overused and has therefore become meaningless at times. The following qualities, I believe, are the ones that qualify an individual to be a true master teacher."

- "A Master teacher has years of study and experience under his/her belt. Study and experience have to be earned. These are processes that by their very nature imply years of dedication to a certain area of expertise. Of course we can debate about how many years this takes: ten, twenty, thirty? I could not tell you, but certainly not two, three, or five by any stretch of the imagination. On top of studying the method, a master teacher embodies the philosophy of Pilates teachings and what these mean. Master teachers integrate these into each cell of their bodies. They walk, talk, and breathe them; they practice.

- "A Master teacher also has to have excellent skill. He or she should have achieved the absolute highest level of practice in the method at some point in their lives. Achieving skill is a journey; it makes you realize that when you reach your goal, it is so that you can start at the beginning again with more understanding and purpose. You must reach the highest level of the work to then go back and focus on the most basic and simple exercises, like a pelvic curl, and find deeper meaning and potential in them.

A master teacher is not only a good teacher, but also a unique teacher and a unique practitioner. What makes the person unique is often intangible, but they seem to stand out as 'jewels in the crown' and are considered as such by their peers.

- "A Master teacher should also have unique human qualities. Being able to transcend the ego, transcend politics in order to share expertise with humility. These teachers are not scared of sharing, changing and, most importantly, of failing. I believe we need to be less rigid, more flexible in our approaches and beliefs, particularly if we see the direction of our work as sometimes having negative repercussions.

- "This willingness to accept change brings me to my next point: a master teacher is always also a student. If you lose the passion for learning, then you need to stop teaching immediately. I visit courses and listen to lectures at conferences regularly and I can tell immediately if someone has stopped learning. To me, this means that they cannot be a master teacher. Teachers should also be in shape; we cannot teach something like Pilates at a high level and look like we have not done a session in six months. Master teachers are unique people, in constant search of ideals, trying to embody their philosophies into their lives and always striving to be better. Only then are they credible."

A master teacher, then, combines experience, skill, empathy, and humility, and always seeks to learn more.

Integrating research-based findings into the creation a Pilates-adapted method has been the primary goal of Moira and Lindsay Merrithew at Stott Pilates. Although Moira was trained by one of Pilates' students, Romana Krysanowska, she took her teaching a step further in order to integrate scientific information into her programs. "Romana is a charismatic woman and has a lot to offer in terms of what she was taught by Joseph Pilates," Moira says. "For us at Stott however, research-based knowledge from physical therapists and medical professionals has been key when developing our approach."

How Do You Find a Mentor? Start Looking. . .

When I opened my studio in Germany, there were only three small studios in town. One year later, there seemed to be courses, classes, and studios popping up at every corner. Some will survive (the good ones!), some will not. If a studio has been around for a long time, you can almost guarantee that there is a mentor in that building.

And we, the trainers, need to go and find out who it is and what he or she does. A mentor is an absolute must for anyone in the bodywork community. We need individuals who we can trust in order to discuss conflicts, seek counsel, and grow. This work is all about communion. Without communion, there can be no learning; and without learning, there cannot be any transformation.

A mentor provides the opportunity for development for us, the trainers, and simultaneously teaches us what will be expected of us in the future, when we hopefully become mentors ourselves.

Mentorship Hunt

There are several superb advantages in store when you embark on a mentorship hunt.

1. Learn something new.

No matter how long you have been in the business, hearing the same things phrased another way is refreshing and inspiring. Usually, you will pick up an exercise, a new image, a verbal cue, or some good anatomical information.

If you are lucky, you may get some personal corrections that are helpful and provide a new incentive for improvement. If you are really lucky, you will come out feeling happy, which is what you would like your clients to feel like when they leave you.

2. Witness a different studio environment.

Studios have their own personalities, and this very element will directly relate to the clientele in the studio and the trainers who are working there.

Indirect lighting, background music, and a tea kitchen are fundamental elements for me to have; others may like it more "clean" and less homey. Whatever it is, whether it is learning more about your likes or your dislikes, taking class at a different studio gives you information for the future.

3. Meet a different clientele.

Most of the time, your personality, age, gender, and special interests will influence the types of clients with whom you work. If you work in only one studio, referrals will soon create a client base of individuals who are somehow related to one another.

Visiting a different studio opens up a lot of opportunity for identifying other markets and meeting people from different social groups who have an interest in Pilates.

Take notes! What is the male/female ratio, what kind of jobs do these individuals do, which interests do they pursue, what are their family histories, do they have injuries?

Imagine that you are a botanist on an exploration mission just tapping into an unknown forest of trees from a new species. This population likes Pilates, spends money on it, and has found just what they need, but not from you.

4. Establish credibility.

A well-known quote says: "If you take it from one it's plagiarism; if you take it from two it's research."

Take "it" from many more than two; even if the studio is your direct competitor, there is nothing they can really say to deter you from taking class there if you are polite, open, and honest about your willingness to learn. Exposing yourself to criticism gives you the "learner's edge," and it's all to your advantage.

Be consistent, though: just showing up once will not give you a good reputation. Support your Pilates community by investing in it. The most profitable way to invest is to take class.

5. Create opportunity for friendship.

In my experience, people in the Pilates community are incredibly good-willed, generous, and kind. Nobody feels good when threatened, however, and therefore we have an obligation to nurture our market through acknowledgement of other instructors and their creative work. Doing this creates a fertile soil for growing friendships, thus generating support and goodwill.

6. Build new job markets.

One other positive element of taking class is that you will invariably be asked to substitute teach when the instructor has an emergency.

Try to do him or her the favor if you can. It helps the other instructor out and creates a platform in which you can shine. Always remember to retreat gracefully by acknowledging the original teacher. Never, ever, hand out your contact information.

If they want you, they will find you.

I would like to thank those who have learned from Mr. Pilates himself and spent their lifetimes mentoring many generations of teachers:

Mary Bowen, Ron Fletcher, Robert Fitzgerald, Eve Gentry Kathy Grant, Romana Kryzanowska, Mary Pilates-LeRich, Hannah Sackmerda, Lolita San Miguel, Bob Seed, and Carola Trier:

Bravo and Thank You!

10
Future Opportunity:
Mastering and Expanding Our Craft

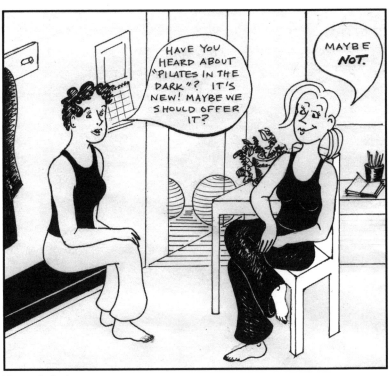

Pilates in the Dark

am tired of paying for workshops that package Pilates exercises into marketable entities by using different pieces of equipment. Don't get me wrong—variety is fun and adds color to our programs, but it can also go a little too far.

We have many different options here: balance on the ball, use the roller, squeeze the fitness circle, pull the flex-band, get challenged on the BOSU. Do Pilates standing up or lying down, try it in the heat or even in the cold, try it early morning or late at night—and, the most hilarious one of all—try it in the DARK! This is not a joke; they honestly offer this at a local Michigan gym. Needless to say, I do not teach it.

Pilates in the dark? What is the point of that, you may ask. At least I was admittedly intrigued, so I made a point of calling. The enlightening conversation went as follows:

Gym Manager (friendly, empowered, male): "Name of Gym, how can I help you?"

Niki (Pilates trainer in disguise, light voice with giggling undertone, female): "Good morning, I read about your Pilates in the dark classes in your brochure. Can you tell me a little bit more about this, since I have taken many Pilates classes, but never in the dark?

Gym Manager (serious, empowered, patronizing): "Pilates is actually always done in the dark. With the lights off, we can let go of our inhibitions and get in touch with our bodies. This is the true meaning of body-mind fitness. Your mind can let go of the worries related to your physical appearance (Niki's thought: Now, that's a nice thing to say to a potential client!) so you can exercise in a carefree state of mind."

Aha! In a way I am glad that some people pay money for exercising in the dark. Now I can feel even better about offering natural light AND candles for coziness in my studio.

$39.95!

Now that Pilates is an industry, competition is a reality. If you do a

Pilates certification search on the Internet, you come up with 60,000 hits. Everybody is fighting for a share of the market. Kevin Bowen, president of the PMA, told me that now you can buy a Pilates certificate for $39.95 over the internet. Everybody can hang a sign on their doors and claim that they are qualified to do the job! I could not believe it.

These developments have created an immediate and desperate need for trainers, the education of whom is a matter of controversy in the Pilates world. Certification programs range from very thorough, in-depth course work with required 800 hours of apprenticeship, anatomy, special populations courses, and exams, to allowing trainers to be certified in two days.

Choosing any educational path is dependent on many variables, such as prior experience in the field of bodywork, time restrictions, and financial considerations.

I understand that the need for trainers encourages many people from "related" movement professions to look into a certification program; I also understand that not everybody is able to invest money and about two years of time and effort into a well-rounded Pilates education. What I don't understand is how some people assume that they are fit to teach after a weekend workshop. This is the fault of the expedited certification organizations—offering courses that dilute the work down to ten exercises. Taking a workshop for one's own development is fine, but thinking that this translates into expertise is questionable. Most importantly, a method only works well in its entirety, with the full spectrum of possibilities explored.

Pilates training has such a large body of work to master and learn. If we focus exclusively on the vast number of exercises and the different types of equipment that are at our disposal, this can keep us busy for a year. On top of that, we have anatomical information and knowledge about special needs populations to master. Since Pilates has such a great reputation for rehabilitation, we have enormous responsibility to perform the teacher's role well.

In order to protect the work, we need a new approach to the certification process. During his address at the Polestar conference in Miami, Kevin Bowen, president of the Pilates Method Alliance, described the PMA's view on the direction the Pilates profession is going. "There is a definite climate change in the air," he said. "Fitness is under a lot of scrutiny from the federal government due to the plethora of injuries that have been inflicted on clients from poorly taught personal trainers. Soon fitness institutions will require employers to only hire trainers who hold certifications that are accredited by NOCA. Right now, out of the hundreds of certifying organizations, only four are accredited."

In America, NCCA (National Commission for Certifying Agencies) and NOCA (National Organization for Competency Assurance) are responsible for regulating certifications according to a set of standards put in place my the American Psychological Association and the US Equal Employment Opportunity. The NCCA accreditation serves as a benchmark for how organizations should conduct certification, and as a fitness organization, you have to meet those standards to become accredited. In order to determine which elements are important to be tested for a given profession, there is NOCA. They gather information on the latest trends and issues of concern to practitioners and organizations focused on certification, licensure, and human resources development.

As Pilates teachers, we are in "la la" land: we are not recognized, our tests are all different depending on the organization administering them, and our tests do not conform to any psychometric standard. We are also not recognized by NOCA, which is one of the reasons why recognition is the PMA's number-one priority right now.

Kevin Bowen and his staff at PMA are hard at work to develop and hopefully establish Pilates as a legal profession in the next three years. The cost of achieving this is astronomical: $300,000!

Will we have to take another test? The answer is yes.

A test is small price to pay for what is to be gained. Once a test is set in place and our job is recognized by law, we could not only have legal coverage, but possibly health insurance and retirement plans. We will not be swimming in the same pool with thousands of other people who have undefined job categories, but we would have a profession in its own right. By joining the PMA as members, we are investing in our future.

While we wait for all of these great things to happen, the issue of continuing education offers many options.

Unless we want to keep taking courses from our certifying organization, a good way to use our continuing education budget is to attend a conference. It is a little expensive due to the traveling and accommodation costs, but it is a truly wonderful experience that is well worth paying for.

The individuals sharing the stage at these levels are few and they are outstanding. Not only will their knowledge amaze you; usually they are also pretty darn good at presenting their life philosophies. You will leave inspired, especially if routine and daily life have been running you down lately, and get a much-needed boost of energy.

Conferences are generally organized by large certifying organization, and sometimes by independent organizers. The PMA hosts a yearly conference in which the first-generation teachers are featured and teach. The Body Mind Spirit conference in Santa Clara is probably the largest in the USA, covering not only Pilates, but Gyrotonic and Yoga as well.

Then there are conferences or meetings organized by individual organizations that are primarily geared toward developing their own teachers, such as the Development Weekends at Body Control Pilates in the U.K. or the Polestar conference in Miami.

Lynne Robinson and her husband Leigh can't even keep up with the demand. They are now running four workshops per year and the thirst for knowledge of their teachers is endless. These gatherings are great. You meet people who do the same thing in different countries of the world, experience new teachers, and network. I picked up quite a few teaching gigs after attending my first conference a few years ago and ran into a mentor as well.

Now that we know what to look for in the teacher, there are more hoops to jump through. Pilates is not only enjoying growth, but is also being adapted to many different populations. Body Control Pilates is offering many more certification courses in Applied Pilates (such as Pilates for children and equine Pilates) and "focus days" on topics such as pregnancy, osteoporosis, and biomechanics. Then there is yogilates, clinical Pilates, athletic Pilates, standing Pilates, and Pilates communication (my baby!!). Are we building niches to make the method more accessible and broaden the scope of our activities? Is this good or bad? What are the problems with these specialty courses?

Let's assume the following scenario:

Somebody studies and teaches Pilates for ten years. Is a physical therapist or doctor who completes a weekend course a better or an equal teacher? Does previous training in another related discipline allow people to jump ahead and claim expertise?

Here, as you can imagine, the opinions are divided.

Brent Anderson at Polestar built a thriving rehabilitation center by bringing Pilates to physical therapists. A physical therapist himself, to Brent it made sense to bring what he knew to his own professional community. Brent supports and encourages research on Pilates and put the method on the map for physical therapists and dance medicine researchers.

Polestar also has a very people-friendly workshop, where teachers can visit the Miami facility for week at the low cost of $250 and witness the application of Pilates for rehabilitation. "Anybody is welcome," Brent says. "We encourage people with broad interests to explore these with us."

Here is the other side of the coin. There are economic reasons behind wanting to bring the medical community onto our side. We want them to understand what we do and endorse the method. They, however, are very unlikely to put in the time and money into a full certification. So, we compromise, teaching them a little and handing out a certification on the grounds of previous training.

These people then go out and lead workshops on Pilates because they have "MD" or "PT" after their names, while those who studied and are "just" dancers or "just" fitness instructors or "just" housewives (or whatever it is that we did before Pilates) feel a little baffled.

What a dilemma. . .now what? Rael Isacowitz has thoughts on this—strong ones:

"Whatever you do, you have to study Pilates first and not just use it as a specialization vehicle for another line of work," he says. "By doing so, you are giving away the essence and authenticity of it all."

There is more.

"My point is that in two days, whether you are a physical therapist or not, you know nothing about Pilates—you don't even know what you don't know." Rael continues, "We are placing PT's and Doctors onto a pedestal that has no foundation, just to get them on our side. I have been teaching PT's for years. Some are very talented; some, however, know nothing about functional anatomy and even less about movement. This is a method in its own right, not a tag line. As such, it deserves to be studied seriously."

Leadership Development

There is another aspect to personal development that is as yet little explored. I was wondering if there are any plans to monitor and foster leadership in the teacher community. In other words, once I have finished my exam and am certified, what are my career options with my organization? Do I get evaluated and rewarded for my work? What other activities are possible if running a studio successfully does not satisfy me in the long run?

In the future, could Pilates become an athletic discipline, a performance art, a teaching career, or a research area? And would such a development not allow the different people choosing one or more areas of study to be rewarded for things at which they excel?

It seems to me that creating focus within Pilates training would create a solid base for the plan ahead to become a legal profession. It would also give us opportunity as a community to foster our interest and expand our field of action. We really need to focus our teaching outreach on children. It is great for them and broadens our scope. Moira Merrithew, for example, taught a successful course to Canadian highschoolers, who are crazy about hockey. They loved it, especially the guys who kept coming back for more and more! Kids like sports or dance. That's the way to "get" them.

1. Pilates as Athletic Discipline

The advanced work in Pilates is absolutely athletic! I would think that anybody who has seen it performed would agree with that. It is vigorous and gymnastic, and requires very advanced levels of control, physical fitness, and practice. On the downside, we hardly get to experience it unless we study daily for years. Building up the strength and flexibility to sustain a full advanced workout is no easy task. For my part, I would enjoy watching Pilatistas who have reached this level of skill.

Some organizations are beginning to launch Pilates routines in a competition format, much like dance or gymnastic competitions. Maybe this development would open Pilates to the younger generations. Rehabilitation is a good motivator for people with functional problems. These people tend to be older. We are not going to make Pilates for kids cool by raving about their improved future health. Who cares! They don't.

2. Pilates as Performance

Pilates also has artistic qualities to it, like that we see when dancers "flow" from one exercise into the next. Elizabeth Larkam's group regularly performs choreographed pieces on the Pilates equipment, which are set to music. Again, the activities could broaden the understanding of Pilates by taking it into the "hobby" realm of things. People love to move to music, so why not combine the skill of learning Pilates with the enjoyment of moving to the beat?

3. Pilates as a Teaching Career

Some humans are just "born" to teach. They love imparting knowledge and finding new avenues of understanding. These should be the true master teachers, the ones who are chosen to be instructor trainers and will be featured in videos, books, and conferences. They could assume leadership roles in terms of bringing Pilates into schools and into health programs. They are articulate, educated, connected, and respected.

4. Pilates and Research

Researchers are people who like to build knowledge through scientific experimentation. Pilates researchers could explore how Pilates work can help children and people with disabilities, or how it can enhance learning and concentration. These researchers provide scientific backup for the teachers and discover new possibilities for the work in order to create a solid foundation for the Pilates future.

These ideas are not unreasonable. They are part of the classic division of skills that every business that experiences incredible growth in a short period of time needs to address. We cannot be good at everything, but we can create and appreciate development opportunities for separate areas of knowledge.

Reinventing mind-body fitness in the year 2004?

Everything is possible, but not in the dark. . .please.

11

Do You Know These People?

The Pilates Alibists

- Have a hard time focusing because they do not really like to work out and use Pilates as an "alibi"
- Ask millions of questions but only does a third of the exercises
- Would love to include "Talking on the Phone" in the repertory of Pilates exercises
- Look at the clock many times throughout the session
- Compliment you on your outfit in order to divert from moving
- Are unhappy with their physical appearances because the exercises are (obviously) not working. These are the clients who run into the studio waving their arms frantically in order to show you that they have no triceps (the "Hello" muscles)

ⓘ Mostly women, very nice people, lack motivation.

⚒ You need to create rewards and drag them through the workout ("Come on: two more, one more, well done!").

High Maintenance, hard work for us!

The Pilates Analysts

- Love to analyze what they do; Brain vs. Body is the issue here

- Must know everything about the exercises

    o   What is it for?

    o   Where should I feel this?

    o   Which muscles are involved?

    o   What is the daily application?

- Either need all the information to brag in front of their friends or are just analytical, interested individuals

- A good way for new trainers to practice anatomy (and get quizzed on it!)

ⓘ Mostly men, intense personalities, motivated, on time.

✗ If you have lots of energy, do the talking and explaining. On an off day, just make the workout difficult to shut them up. They will love you for it.

💥 Medium Maintenance, folks to look forward to teaching.

The Pilates Sufferers

- Love to Suffer

- Always in pain

- Never in pain the in same places as the week before

- Constant complaining and craving modifications to feel listened to

- They say they "don't feel anything"

- They will stay with you forever

ⓘ Mostly women. Usually a little late, but also late to leave. Never schedule the Analyst after the Sufferer!

✖ Remember to ask about last week's injury, make sure that this week's injury is not a "real" one, and get on with the work.

✴ High Maintenance, very loyal!

The Pilates Cosmopolitans

- "Seen it all, done it all" approach

- High body awareness

- Fit and willing to learn

- Will assess your performance in every session, so avoid "robot" tone of voice when queuing the exercises—they will spot this immediately

- Only as loyal to you as you are to them. It is not enough to provide a good workout, they want more: information, challenge, daily custom-made workout

ⓘ Women and Men. On time, rarely cancel, know their schedule months ahead of time and will make sure they book in with you. They take it badly if you have to cancel on them!

✖ Information is key. They feel best when you provide a challenging workout and add stimulating intellectual information.

✸ High Maintenance, but it's worth it!

The Pilates Muscle Fanatics

- Train 4 times per week (at least!)

- Want more spring load. These are the clients who ask you about wrapping weights around their legs for "extra" challenge

- Do not really understand the work (that's why they need more springs to keep coming back!)

- They never admit that Pilates is hard (only when they are close to death because you have provided them with a full advanced workout)

- You have to make them sweat for them to be happy

ⓘ Women and men. On time, but very busy people. They change their appointments five times out of ten.

✗ Alternate workouts: one day you do a gym-like session with lots of springs, the next time you do mat (which they loathe!).

✖ Medium Maintenance, great to work with.

The Pilates Spartans

- Give 100% every time
- Stone faced or tensed facial expression
- They simply refuse to breathe
- They will not tell you that they are in pain, even though you can see it from a mile away
- They will do what you say and come back because they can feel relief. You have to find ways to trick them into talking–ask about their hobbies and how pain affects them (be prepared to stay for hours. . .)
- Teach them that relaxing is good for them!

ⓘ Mostly Men. On time, go-getters, usually very tight musculature.

⚒ The more you breathe loudly to encourage them, the less they will follow your example. (By this time we sound hideous and have turned into a puffing Locomotive.)

✷ Low Maintenance, great people!

The Super Pilatistas

- Give 300% every time

- Always in a good mood

- Mostly athletes and sports people, high achievers

- Will remember exercises (and we are very grateful for that!)

- They will be with you all the way—stretch their limits and your own

ⓘ Women and Men. On time, go-getters, no complaints. You have to make sure you ask about injuries because they will not tell you.

✘ Alternate workouts and pieces of equipment as well as speed and pace.

✼ Low Maintenance, Pilates instructor heaven!

References

American College of Obstetricians and Gynecologists. "Sexuality and Sexual Problems." http://www.medem.com/medlb/article_detaillb.cfm?article_ID=ZZZ7P2WBT7C&sub_cat=2004

Fawcett, Nichole. "Patching up low libido: Study examines testosterone in women." University of Michigan Press Release. http://www.med.umich.edu/opm/newspage/2004/hmlowlibido.htm

Foley, Sally, Sally Kope, and Dennis Sugrue. *Sex Matters for Women: A Complete Guide to Taking Care of Your Sexual Self.* New York: Guildford Press, 2002.

Franklin, Eric. *Pelvic Power for Men and Women: Mind/Body Exercises for Strength, Flexibility, Posture, and Balance.* New Jersey: Elysian Editions, 2002.

Gardner, Howard. *Frames of Mind: The Theory of Multiple Intelligences.* New York: Basic Books, 1983.

Graham, Kathy. "Running ahead: Enhancing teacher commitment," *Journal of Physical Education, Recreation and Dance* 67 (1996).

Hughes, Patricia, and Ian Kerr. "Transference and countertransference in communication between doctor and patient," *Advances in Psychiatric Treatment* 6 (2000): 57 – 64.

Human Factors and Ergonomics Society of Australia. www.ergonomics.org.au/erginfoprac.html

Knodt, Gerrit. *Developing Excellent People Managers: A Road Less Traveled.* Philadelphia: Xllibris Corporation, 2002.

Larkin, Geri. *Building a Business the Buddhist Way: A Practitioner's Guidebook.* Berkeley: Celestial Arts, 1999.

. *Tap Dancing in Zen.* Berkeley: Celestial Arts, 2000.

McIntosh, Nina. *The Educated Heart: Professional Guidelines for Massage Therapists, Bodyworkers and Movement Teachers.* Tennessee: Decatur Bainbridge Press, 1999.

National Commission for Certifying Agencies (NCAA) Accreditation Information.
http://www.noca.org/ncca/accreditation.htm

National Institute of Health, The. "Dietary Supplements: Vitamin D." http://www.cc.nih.gov/ccc/supplements/vitd.html

Peters, Joan. *When Mothers Work: Loving Our Children Without Sacrificing Ourselves*. Boston: Perseus Book Group, 1998.

Pilates, Joseph, Judd Robbins, and William Miller. *Pilates' Return to Life Through Contrology*. Incline Village, NV: Presentation Dynamics, 1998.

Project SUMIT: Theory of Multiple Intelligences.
http://www.pz.harvard.edu/SUMIT.html

Rubin, Harriet. *Soloing: Realizing Your Life's Ambition*. New York: HarperBusiness, 1999.

Sorgen, Carol. "To stay healthy...Make friends," *Medscape Health for Consumers* (2001).
http://www.health.medscape.com/viewarticle/
411465.html

Stonington, J. "Let the Sun Shine," *Natural Family Online Newsletter*.
http://www.naturalfamilyonline.com/NH/20044_sunshine
.htm

Stanley, Lawrence E. "About the Name Pilates."
http://www.pilatesbodytrends.com/products/pilates/
pilname.html

Sternberg, Robert. "Identifying and Developing Creative Giftedness," *Roper Review* 23, no. 2 (2000).

Taylor, Glenda. *Aromatherapy for Relaxation, Beauty, and Good Health.* New York: William Morrow and Company, 2000.

Vincent, Lawerence. *Competing with the Sylph: The Quest for the Perfect Dance Body.* New Jersey: Princeton Books, 1989.

Windsor, Mari, and Mark Laska. *The Pilates Powerhouse.* Boston: Perseus Books.

Wood, Julia. *Relational Communication: Continuity and Change in Personal Relationships.* Belmont: Wadsworth Publishing Company, 2000.

Acknowledgment

Who would ever have thought that I could write a book?

This was no lonesome experience; in fact, without so many amazing people who are part of my life, I would never have finished it. We discussed endlessly: on the phone, at dinner, at lunch, at breakfast, during Pilates sessions, at our favorite coffee shop, Eastern Accents, in bed, on a sailboat, on planes, in cars!

The settings of these conversations were in several countries: England, Germany, Italy, Greece, South Africa, and the United States. It sometimes felt like every section and every chapter were inspired by and shared with a herd of likeminded people!

Thank you, from the bottom of my heart, to my Ann Arbor family and core supporters of this project:

To George Evans, for allowing me to cover his living room with huge Post-its on Logokinesis last October—the foundation for this book.

To sculptor, painter, and friend Susan Byrnes. You thought you were done with dance. . .and now this! I will trade my body parts in exchange for your brilliant comics forever!

To the only person who truly doesn't speak "business" but always looks at relationships: Claudette Jocelyn Stern. What would I do without your counsel? Kick in the butt? Inspiring postcards and poems? Merci for making me one step closer to becoming a "diva with empathy!"

To Holly Furgason, for beautiful graphic design, publishing insights, and friendship, and for leaving me speechless by observing your talent and beauty. Some people just have it all...

To Amy Burke. A night on the town in San Francisco brought us together under unusual circumstances. How you navigated through my quadrilingual manuscript I do not know—thank you for everything.

To my family, especially Bernadette Conraths and Gerrit Knodt, who helped along the way with comments and human resource knowledge, I owe thanks for constant support for my millions of projects.

In the Pilates field, I would like to express gratitude and much love for Sylvia Rohmann, Aimee McDonald, Kornelia Ritterpusch, Bridget Montague, John Sealey, Carolyne Anthony, Philip Madrid—your voices are in this book!

To the founders of the Pilates corporations represented in this book, I want to extend my deepest thanks! Although I was scared stiff when I approached all of you, your willingness to share has been amazing. Brent Anderson, Kevin Bowen, Rael Isacowitz, Elizabeth Larkam, Lynne Robinson, and Moira and Lindsay Merrithew—you rock!

To Nancy Hodari, Eva Powers, Trent McEntire, Donna Gambino, Barbara Basset, and all the teachers I have spoken to for peer review and feedback: Bravo!

To my parents, Hans and Karin Conraths. Thank you for letting me dance.

To Jens Lange. . .what can I say? I love you.

To my clients. The biggest applause of all goes to you. Without you, there would be no book.

Contact Information

The Alderley Pilates Studio
Peter and Jan Bowen
Monks Heath Hall
Nether Alderley
Cheshire SK11 9SU
United Kingdom
Phone: +44 1625 860475
Email: alderleypilates@btconnect.com

Body Arts and Science International
Rael Isacowitz, MA
Founder and Director
485 E. 17th Street, Suite 650
Costa Mesa, CA 92627
USA
Phone: +1 949 574 1343
Fax: +1 949 642 8139
Email: info@basipilates.com
Web: www.basipilates.com

Body Control Pilates Group
6 Langley Street
London WC2H 9JA
United Kingdom
Phone: +44 207 379 3734
Fax: +44 207 379 7551
Web: www.bodycontrolpilates.com

The Center for Women's Fitness
Carolyne Anthony, Director
2371 Delaware Drive
Ann Arbor, MI 48103
USA
Phone: +1 734 668 4077

Core Grace Pilates
Khita Whyatt
211 S. 4th Avenue, Suite 1B
Ann Arbor, MI 48104
USA
Phone: +1 734 913 9046
Web: www.coregracepilates.com

Creative Body Engineering
Philip Madrid
10109 Baldwin Ave
Albuquerque, NM 87112
USA
Phone: +1 505 332 3562

Equilibrium: Mind-Body Fitness
A Stott Pilates Licensed Certification Center
Nancy Hodari, Director
Eva Powers, MA, Associate Professor, Wayne State University
Kim Dunleavy, MS, PT, OCS
6405 Telegraph, Building G
Bloomfield Medical Village
Bloomfield Hills, MI 48301
USA
Phone: +1 248 723 6500
Email: Nancy@equilibriumstudio.com

Franklin Methode Institut
Brunnenstrasse 1
86106 Usta
Switzerland
Phone: +41 43 399 0603
Fax: +41 43 399 0604

Gyrotonic Expansion System
134 Dingmans Ct.
Dingmans Ferry, PA 18328
USA
Phone: +1 570 828 0003
Email: info@gyrotonic.com
Web: www.gyrotonic.com

InterContext s.p.r.l.
Gerrit Knodt, Senior Partner
Goellesheimer Weg 27
53343 Wachtberg
Germany
Phone: +49 228 28 4992
Email: Gerrit.Knodt@skynet.be
Web: www.inter-context.com

Interkinetic Creative Group
Holly Furgason
San Francisco, CA
USA
Email: info@ikcgroup.com
Web: www.ikcgroup.com

McEntire Workout Method
Trent McEntire, Program Director
438 Main Street, Suite 207
Rochester, MI 48307
USA
Phone: +1 248 651 5567 or toll free +1 866 373 8600
Email: trent@mcentiremethod.com
Web: www.mcentiremethod.com

Movement Center
Aimee McDonald & Nicola Conraths-Lange
201 East Liberty Street, Suite 6
Ann Arbor, MI 48104
USA
Web: www.movement-center.com

Namasta—North American Studio Alliance
2313 Hastings Drive
Belmont, CA 94002
USA
Phone: +1 877 626 2782
Web: www.namasta.com

Pilates & Beyond
Elizabeth Larkam, Director
Western Athletic Clubs
One Lombard Street
San Francisco, CA 94111
USA
Phone: +1 415 901 9310
Email: elarkam@wac-clubs.com

Pilates Forms
Sylvia Rohmann
Brahmsallee 16
20144 Hamburg
Germany
Email: sylvia.rohmann@freenet.de

Pilates Method Alliance
P.O.Box 370906
Miami, FL 33137
USA
Phone: +1 866 573 4945
Fax: +1 305 573 4461
Email: info@pilatesmethodalliance.org
Web: www.pilatesmethodalliance.org

Polestar Pilates Education LLC
International Headquarters
12380 SW 82 Avenue
Miami, FL 33156
USA
Phone: +1 305 666 0037 or toll free +1 800 387 3651
Web: www.polestarpilates.com

Lindsay & Moira Merrithew, Co-founders
Stott Pilates
2200 Yonge Street, Suite 500
Toronto, ON M4S 2C6
Canada
Phone: +1 416-482-4050 or toll free +1 800 910 0001
Fax: +1 416 482 2742
Email: info@stottpilates.com
Web: www.stottpilates.com

Studio für Körperbewusstsein
Kornelia Ritterpusch
Grindelhof 89, Hs.9, Garten
20146 Hamburg
Germany
Phone: +49 40 410 7273
Fax: +49 404 136 3417
Email: Kornelia@studiofuerkoerperbewusstsein.de